EACH YEAR AMERICANS SPEND WELL OVER A BILLION DOLLARS ON VITAMIN AND MINERAL SUPPLEMENTS. ARE YOU SPENDING TOO MUCH —OR TOO LITTLE? ARE YOU TAKING THE RIGHT VITAMINS FOR YOUR BODY AND LIFESTYLE?

THE VITAMIN BOOK gives you all the facts about the nutrients you need, and answers today's most-asked questions:

- Is it possible to get all the nutrients necessary for good health from the food you eat?

- When are supplements helpful, which ones should you buy, and how many should you take?

- What are the facts about vitamin megadoses—can they prevent and even cure disease?

- Do megadoses actually do more harm than good?

THE VITAMIN BOOK

A No-Nonsense Consumer Guide

**by Harold M. Silverman, Pharm.D.,
Joseph A. Romano, Pharm.D.
and Gary Elmer, Ph.D.**

BANTAM BOOKS
NEW YORK · TORONTO · LONDON · SYDNEY · AUCKLAND

For Barbara, Melissa, and Jennifer Silverman,
Linda, Nicholas Joseph, and Christine Dianne Romano
and Joan Elmer

THE VITAMIN BOOK: A NO-NONSENSE CONSUMER GUIDE
A Bantam Book / August 1985

ISBN 0-553-27435-X

Published simultaneously in the United States and Canada

Bantam Books are published by Bantam Books, a division of Bantam Doubleday Dell Publishing Group, Inc. Its trademark, consisting of the words "Bantam Books" and the portrayal of a rooster, is Registered in U.S. Patent and Trademark Office and in other countries. Marca Registrada. Bantam Books, 1540 Broadway, New York, New York 10036.

PRINTED IN THE UNITED STATES OF AMERICA

O   20 19 18

Contents

PART III
MINERAL PROFILES

PART IV
VITAMIN, MINERAL, AND DRUG INTERACTIONS 271

Tables

Introduction

Vitamins and minerals are big business. Each year, Americans spend well over a billion dollars on vitamin and mineral supplements, much of which is probably unnecessary. Vitamins are also one of the hottest topics in today's media. Every day we read or hear about a new cancer cure, miracle diet, health plan, or other heretofore unknown use for a vitamin, mineral, or vitamin–mineral combination. What *are* these miracle drugs, these sources of eternal youth, beauty, and sexual prowess, these cures for the diseases that plague our lives? Are they really so miraculous?

Experts agree that vitamins and minerals are needed to prevent some deficiency conditions, among them a few life-threatening deficiency diseases. There is sharp disagreement, though, on how to get these vitamins into your body. Some people believe that you can get everything you need by eating a "balanced" diet. Others feel that today's fast-paced lifestyle dictates the use of vitamin and mineral supplements to make certain you get everything you need. Still others believe that megadoses of vitamins and/or minerals are the key to preventing and treating (or even curing!) a whole host of diseases. Health authorities generally feel that the concept of treating disease with megavitamin therapy has no merit. But many consumer advocates, the health food industry, and a small but vocal group of doctors believe everyone should take supplements and that megadoses are a cure-all approach to treating disease.

Are vitamins and minerals the essence of life that has been kept hidden away from us? Unfortunately, as consumers, we have had almost no place to go for straightforward, simple answers to the questions we most want answered about vitamin and mineral supplements. Most consumer-oriented books on the subject are written by vitamin advocates and offer a hard-sell approach. Arguments in these works are often based on scanty factual data and offer nonscientific approaches to selecting the vitamins and minerals you need to maintain your health.

Information in *The Vitamin Book*, on the other hand, has been gleaned from hundreds of scientific publications. We have tried to dispel the myths, mysteries, and untruths commonly associated with vitamins and minerals. Here you will learn what vitamins and minerals are, where they work in your body, when you need them, what they can do for you, how much to take, and how to select a vitamin and/or mineral preparation from the hundreds that line the shelves of your health food store, pharmacy, or vitamin shop.

We believe that many, but not all, people will benefit by taking supplemental vitamins and/or minerals; that vitamins are not particularly harmful, except when taken in unusually large doses, at which point they are not being used for their effect as vitamins but as drugs to modify a disease, with the potential for serious side effects. So far, vitamin supplements have dramatically influenced the course of few single diseases, although chemical derivatives of some vitamins have proved to be of great therapeutic value for some illnesses. Unfortunately, you can't get the same effects by using the vitamin itself.

We believe that future research will lead to ways in which vitamins can be of some benefit *as a part of* the treatment of diseases such as cancer, heart disease, and the common cold. But until that information becomes available, indiscriminate use of vitamins and minerals may do us more harm than good.

In the final analysis, only you can determine how helpful this book will be. Use the information on the pages that follow to

make reasonable decisions about the vitamins you and your family use as part of your plan to achieve and maintain good health.

HAROLD M. SILVERMAN, Pharm.D.
JOSEPH A. ROMANO, Pharm.D.
GARY ELMER, Ph.D.

Part I

SHOULD YOU TAKE
VITAMINS AND MINERALS?

1

What Are Vitamins and Minerals and How Do They Work?

There are some forty different substances known to be essential elements of human nutrition. Of these, thirteen are recognized as vitamins and fifteen are recognized as either essential minerals (needed in large amounts), trace minerals (needed only in small amounts), or electrolytes.

Vitamins

The scientific discovery of vitamins as separate nutrients was launched in the late nineteenth century, when scientists and nutritionists began to examine specific foods already known for centuries to prevent the occurrence of certain diseases: oranges for scurvy, unpolished rice for beriberi and pellagra. Then, in the early twentieth century, Casimir Funk, a Polish biochemist working in London, isolated a crystalline substance from rice polishings and coined the word *vitamine* to describe this "amine" (a kind of chemical structure) which was essential for life. Later it was shown that not all vitamins share the amine structure and the final "e" was dropped, giving us the modern spelling, vitamin.

Research continued through the 1930s and 1940s, when

many of the basic facts about vitamins were discovered. This history of vitamins offers some interesting scientific stories and is associated with several Nobel prizes.

The most recent vitamin and mineral research has been directed toward learning more about their effects on the body and new uses for them. Much of this work has been spurred on by accidental discoveries about possible new uses for vitamins and minerals. However, most of these studies have yielded either no useful information or results that cannot be reproduced by other investigators, rendering their conclusions questionable.

What Is a Vitamin?

Vitamins are essentially substances made by plants with the help of sunlight or by lower forms of life such as bacteria; in a few cases, vitamins can also be created by animals or the human body. They are always combinations of several chemical elements.

Most of our vitamins come from plants, and interestingly, the amount of a vitamin found in a given plant is always the same because the plant always makes just the right amount it needs to stay alive. For example, the average-size orange usually has about 85 mg. of vitamin C. Vitamins found in animal products, such as eggs, are by-products of the plants ingested by the animal or were created by bacteria.

Over the years, scientists have developed three criteria by which a substance can be defined as a vitamin. If one of the three criteria is not satisfied, the substance in question is not considered a vitamin, in the strictest scientific sense:

1. A vitamin is a nutrient required in small amounts for normal body function. With few exceptions, vitamins are not made in the body and must be supplied from an outside source. Even in those few circumstances where vitamins are "made" in the body, the process generally involves an important ingredient from outside the body, such as the bacteria normally found in our intestines.

2. A vitamin must be an organic chemical, that is, every vitamin has at least one carbon atom in its molecular structure. This automatically excludes minerals and other noncarbon-containing substances.

3. There is a specific set of symptoms or disease associated with a deficiency of each vitamin that can be corrected by taking the appropriate amount of that vitamin.

It is unfortunate that advocates of vitamin treatments for illness have used the word *vitamin* improperly. Many of the proposed treatments involve doses of vitamins so far beyond the amounts required for normal nutrition that they are, in fact, no longer vitamins but drugs. Also, many treatments involve substances that do not meet the established criteria for vitamins and are therefore discussed in this book in Part II under "Pseudovitamins." These include PABA, choline, inositol, and other substances that have been labeled vitamins simply in an effort to lend them public credibility.

Pressure from the U.S. Food and Drug Administration has forced the elimination of most pseudovitamins from multivitamin products. Despite the fact that these substances are either abundant in the food we eat or are not needed for daily function, however, they are still available for purchase in any health food store or vitamin center.

How Vitamins Work

Vitamins are chemical gears in the complex machine we call the human body. Each vitamin fits into a different part of the machine, and all of them are necessary for normal body function.

Chemists would call most vitamins cofactors (or catalysts). A cofactor is a substance that helps chemical reactions occur but is not a primary ingredient in the reaction. A rough analogy is the oil in your car's crankcase: although it is an essential ingredient to your automobile engine, it is not a major ingredient in the chemical reaction that makes the engine work. The major ingredients are gasoline, oxygen, and a spark. The oil helps this chemical reaction reach maximum efficiency by keeping all the moving parts of your engine running as smoothly and friction free as possible.

Vitamins perform the same function in the body. For example:

• Vitamin B_1 (thiamin) is a cofactor in the series of chemical reactions that burn carbohydrates (sugars) in the body. Without thiamin, you would not be able to provide sufficient energy for body functions and would die.

• Vitamin B$_2$ (riboflavin) serves as a cofactor in many chemical reactions involving the release of energy from body proteins. For this reason, your riboflavin needs are directly related to the amount of energy you use each day.

• Folic acid serves as a cofactor in one of the chemical reactions that are basic to normal cell division in your body. Cell division is essential to many basic functions, including replacing worn-out body cells with new ones, providing the new cells needed for growth and development, and healing wounds by making new cells.

Is There More Than One Category of Vitamin?

Vitamins fall into two basic categories: those which dissolve in water, and those which dissolve in fat.

Water-Soluble Vitamins

The water-soluble vitamins are: B$_1$ (thiamin), B$_2$ (riboflavin), B$_3$ (nicotinic acid), B$_5$ (pantothenic acid), B$_6$ (pyridoxine), B$_{12}$ (cyanocobalamine), C (ascorbic acid), biotin, and folic acid.

These vitamins can be easily absorbed directly through the gastrointestinal tract into the bloodstream and don't require bile acids or other special substances to assist in this process. Once absorbed, they circulate in body fluids and are available when needed for body function.

Most water-soluble vitamins are not stored in large quantities for long periods of time. Once a certain reserve (the threshold or saturation level) is reached, much of the excess water-soluble vitamin is eliminated from the body via the urine. Therefore, taking more of these vitamins than you need—according to the recommendations discussed in the next chapter—is literally flushing money down the drain and can lead to toxic side effects.

Fat-Soluble Vitamins

The fat-soluble vitamins are A, D, E, and K.

These vitamins are oily substances that require the addition of bile acids, your natural emulsifying agents, to be dissolved in intestinal contents and then absorbed into the bloodstream. The process can be compared to your use of soaps and detergents as emulsifying agents when washing out oily dirt. Since oil and water don't mix, oily dirt cannot be removed by water alone. The detergent allows dirt to emulsify in the wash water, making it easier to remove.

Some fat-soluble vitamins, however, can be purchased in a "water-soluble" form. These products, such as Aquasol A and Aquasol E, consist of vitamin that has been mixed with an emulsifying agent and can be absorbed without the assistance of bile acids.

Once absorbed, the fat-soluble vitamins migrate to their storage sites in body fat. When they are needed in the body, special carrier proteins take the vitamins from their storage areas to the places they are needed.

Because of this storage capability, excessive amounts of some of these vitamins can be retained by the body and result in unpleasant or even hazardous toxicity symptoms. Therefore, taking more of this category of vitamin than you need can be not merely a waste of money, as in the case of water-soluble vitamins, but an investment in unwanted discomfort and inconvenience and can be dangerous to your health.

Each vitamin has a specific action. Some are used more widely than others and are required in larger quantities. The specific functions of each vitamin and its role in human metabolism and function can be found in the individual profiles in Part II of this book.

Minerals

Unlike vitamin research, serious study of the roles of the various minerals in the human body has been carried out mostly during the last two decades. Some minerals have been extensively studied, but many others are not well understood. Minerals such as zinc, nickel, selenium, molybdenum, and manganese are now the subject of research projects all over the world. We believe that the next decade will shed a vast amount of light not only on how these minerals function but also on how they can be used as possible therapeutic agents.

What Is a Mineral?

Minerals are basic elements that have their origin in the soil and, unlike vitamins, cannot be made by living systems. Those that have been found to be essential to body function are calcium, phosphorous, magnesium, iodine, iron, and zinc. Very small amounts of the important trace minerals are copper, chromium, fluorine, manganese, molybdenum, and selenium are also needed by your body. Very little is known about the other trace elements—arsenic, cadmium, cobalt, nickel, silicone, tin, and vanadium. The best guess is that they are required in very small amounts and that even the most nutritionally inadequate diet contains sufficient quantities.

As in the case of vitamins, we get most of our minerals from plants and animal products that contain minerals as a result of the animal's consumption of mineral-rich plant life. However, whereas the vitamin content of a plant is stable, but the mineral content is not. In fact, the amount of any particular mineral in a plant varies dramatically from region to region because of variations in the mineral content of the soil. For instance, iodine is found in much higher concentrations in seaside soils than in those inland. Accordingly, dietary sources of iodine that originate in the sea or areas near the sea are much higher in iodine than those that do not. Plant sources of the mineral usually provide about one-twentieth as much iodine as animal sources that have originated in the sea, such as crab, halibut, perch, and other seafoods. Plants from the sea such as kelp and seaweed provide more than forty thousand times as much iodine per ounce as plants grown inland.

How Minerals Work

In the body, minerals work through a variety of mechanisms. One of the most important roles involves building basic body structure: calcium, phosphorous, magnesium, and fluorine, for example, are major elements in forming bones and teeth. Some minerals are involved with enzyme activity, or they may combine with other chemicals to perform functions that are essential to life: iron, for example, is a basic component of hemoglobin, the chemical contained in red blood cells that carries oxygen throughout our bodies; copper plays a role in the process of building red blood cells and is also found in several different body enzymes; chromium is involved in the metabolism of glucose.

Unlike vitamins, minerals are neither manufactured nor broken down within the body because they are basic elements. However, minerals must combine with vitamins, enzymes, or other body substances to produce their effects. These combinations can be broken down, used up, or eliminated from the body and therefore must be recycled or remade.

Many of the minerals can cause definite adverse effects if you take too much of them. This, in contrast to the vitamins, which are not as often associated with severe adverse effects, has been a natural barrier to the abuse of minerals as vitamins have been abused.

Since there is so much we don't know about the specific functions of minerals in the body, there is considerable speculation as to their possible role. Some people have even promoted the minerals as tools for life extension and treatments for disease, but, although every possibility must be examined, we believe that it is premature to conclude that any of these claims are valid. The specific functions of each mineral and its role in human metabolism and function can be found in the individual profiles in Part III of this book.

Electrolytes

Electrolytes are minerals that serve very specific functions. The most important of these is related to the maintenance of the balance of water within the body: electrolytes encourage or prevent the flow of water across cell membranes by the process of osmosis. Electrolytes also have a role in certain enzyme and chemical reactions and are responsible for transmission of electrical impulses across cell membranes. The specific function of the electrolytes sodium and potassium can be found in Part III of this book. Others are not discussed because only sodium and potassium are widely supplemented.

2

How Many Vitamins and Minerals Do I Need?

There are three official sources of information on average requirements of vitamins and minerals for good nutrition:

• RDA (recommended daily allowances) tables prepared by the Food and Nutrition Board of the National Academy of Sciences
• U.S. RDA tables prepared by the U.S. Food and Drug Administration
• Foreign and international nutrient standards prepared by individual governments or the United Nations Food and Agriculture Organization (FAO) and World Health Organization (WHO)

Of these, the RDA tables will be the most helpful to you. They have been used as the basis for data on vitamin and mineral requirements cited in this book.

RDA Tables

The RDAs were first published in 1941 and are revised every few years to incorporate new knowledge. There is a special committee within the Food and Nutrition Board, called the

Dietary Allowances Committee, whose specific responsibility it is to prepare the RDA tables. The RDAs are used as the basis for many U.S. governmental policy decisions relating to food and nutrition.

Basically, the RDAs are recommendations for average amounts of daily nutrient intake by men, women, boys, and girls in different age groups. Specific recommendations are given for infants, children, teenagers, and adults through age fifty. Everyone over age fifty is grouped into the fifty-one-plus category. The RDAs are meant to *exceed* the actual daily requirement for each person so they can maintain good health. This is done because there is no way of knowing each person's specific nutrient needs, as the actual need for many nutrients is based on personal factors and diet.

How RDAs Are Determined

There are four basic steps to the establishment of an RDA for each nutrient.

First, scientific studies are undertaken and existing information is reviewed to determine the approximate amount of each vitamin and mineral needed to maintain the health of an average person. The daily needs of healthy young males, except for iron where women's needs are considered essential, are used as a criterion and the results then extrapolated into other age groups.

Second, the average amount arrived at from the studies is increased by an additional arbitrary value which the experts feel will meet the requirements of nearly all people in the age/sex group under consideration. This is done to try to ensure that everybody in the specific group receives all the nutrients they need.

The third step involves the addition of another increment to the RDA. This increment is meant to take into account natural differences in the amounts of nutrient absorbed and utilized by different people.

In the case of some nutrients, this difference is directly related to the amount of energy expended each day. Since the B-complex vitamins are involved in the process of generating energy, the more active you are, the more of the B vitamins you need. Some minerals may be needed in larger amounts by the young and growing (iron and calcium), by older people (cal-

Table 1
RECOMMENDED DAILY DIETARY ALLOWANCES
Food and Nutrition Board, National Academy of Sciences-National Research Council
Revised 1980
Designed for the maintenance of good nutrition of practically all healthy people in the U.S.A.[a]

	Age (years)	Weight (kg)	Weight (lbs)	Height (cm)	Height (in)	Protein (g)	Vitamin A (mcg R.E.)[b]	Vitamin D (mcg)[c]	Vitamin E (mg α T.E.)[d]	Vitamin C (mg)	Thiamin (mg)	Riboflavin (mg)	Niacin (mg N.E.)[e]	Vitamin B6 (mg)	Folacin (mcg)	Vitamin B12 (mcg)	Calcium (mg)	Phosphorus (mg)	Magnesium (mg)	Iron (mg)	Zinc (mg)	Iodine (mcg)
Infants	0.0-0.5	6	13	60	24	kg×2.2	420	10	3	35	0.3	0.4	6	0.3	30	0.5	360	240	50	10	3	40
	0.5-1.0	9	20	71	28	kg×2.0	400	10	4	35	0.5	0.6	8	0.6	45	1.5	540	360	70	15	5	50
Children	1-3	13	29	90	35	23	400	10	5	45	0.7	0.8	9	0.9	100	2.0	800	800	150	15	10	70
	4-6	20	44	112	44	30	500	10	6	45	0.9	1.0	11	1.3	200	2.5	800	800	200	10	10	90
	7-10	28	62	132	52	34	700	10	7	45	1.2	1.4	16	1.6	300	3.0	800	800	250	10	10	120
Males	11-14	45	99	157	62	45	1000	10	8	50	1.4	1.6	18	1.8	400	3.0	1200	1200	350	18	15	150
	15-18	66	145	176	69	56	1000	10	10	60	1.4	1.7	18	2.0	400	3.0	1200	1200	400	18	15	150
	19-22	70	154	177	70	56	1000	7.5	10	60	1.5	1.7	19	2.2	400	3.0	800	800	350	10	15	150
	23-50	70	154	178	70	56	1000	5	10	60	1.4	1.6	18	2.2	400	3.0	800	800	350	10	15	150
	51+	70	154	178	70	56	1000	5	10	60	1.2	1.4	16	2.2	400	3.0	800	800	350	10	15	150
Females	11-14	46	101	157	62	46	800	10	8	50	1.1	1.3	15	1.8	400	3.0	1200	1200	300	18	15	150
	15-18	55	120	163	64	46	800	10	8	60	1.1	1.3	14	2.0	400	3.0	1200	1200	300	18	15	150

Age (years)	Weight (kg)	(lbs)	Height (cm)	(in)	Protein (g)	Fat-Soluble Vitamins			Water-Soluble Vitamins							Minerals					
						Vitamin A (mcg R.E.)[b]	Vitamin D (mcg)[c]	Vitamin E (mg α T.E.)[d]	Vitamin C (mg)	Thiamin (mg)	Riboflavin (mg)	Niacin (mg N.E.)	Vitamin B6 (mg)	Folacin (mcg)	Vitamin B12 (mcg)	Calcium (mg)	Phosphorus (mg)	Magnesium (mg)	Iron (mg)	Zinc (mg)	Iodine (mcg)
19-22	55	120	163	64	44	800	7.5	8	60	1.1	1.3	14	2.0	400	3.0	800	800	300	18	15	150
23-50	55	120	163	64	44	800	5	8	60	1.0	1.2	13	2.0	400	3.0	800	800	300	18	15	150
51+	55	120	163	64	44	800	5	8	60	1.0	1.2	13	2.0	400	3.0	800	800	300	10	15	150
Pregnant					+30	+200	+5	+2	+20	+0.4	+0.3	+2	+0.6	+400	+1.0	+400	+400	+150	e	+5	+25
Lactating					+20	+400	+5	+3	+40	+0.5	+0.5	+5	+0.5	+100	+1.0	+400	+400	+150	e	+10	+50

a The allowances are intended to provide for individual variations among most normal persons as they live in the U.S. under normal conditions. Base your diet on a variety of foods to be sure to obtain a variety of other nutrients, human requirements for which are less well defined.

b Vitamin A concentration is expressed in terms of retinol equivalents. See the vitamin A profile for more information.

c 1 mcg. of vitamin D = 400 units.

d Vitamin E potency is expressed in mg. See the vitamin E profile for more information.

e It is impossible to meet the increased iron requirement of pregnancy or breast feeding through diet alone. Therefore, you must take an iron supplement during those times. For more information, see the Iron profile.

18

Estimated Safe and Adequate Daily Intakes of Additional Selected Vitamins and Minerals[a]

	Age (years)	Vitamins			Trace Elements[b]						Electrolytes		
		Vitamin K (mcg)	Biotin (mcg)	Pantothenic Acid (mg)	Copper (mg)	Manganese (mg)	Fluoride (mg)	Chromium (mg)	Selenium (mg)	Molybdenum (mg)	Sodium (mg)	Potassium (mg)	Chloride (mg)
Infants	0–0.5	12	35	2	0.5–0.7	0.5–0.7	0.1–0.5	0.01–0.04	0.01–0.04	0.03–0.06	115–350	350–925	275–700
	0.5–1	10–20	50	3	0.7–1.0	0.7–1.0	0.2–1.0	0.02–0.06	0.02–0.06	0.04–0.08	250–750	425–1275	400–1200
Children	1–3	15–30	65	3	1.0–1.5	1.0–1.5	0.5–1.5	0.02–0.08	0.02–0.08	0.05–0.1	325–975	550–1650	500–1500
and	4–6	20–40	85	3–4	1.5–2.0	1.5–2.0	1.0–2.5	0.03–0.12	0.03–0.12	0.06–0.15	450–1350	775–2325	700–2100
Adolescents	7–10	30–60	120	4–5	2.0–2.5	2.0–3.0	1.5–2.5	0.05–0.2	0.05–0.2	0.1–0.3	600–1800	1000–3000	925–2775
	11+	50–100	100–200	4–7	2.0–3.0	2.5–5.0	1.5–2.5	0.05–0.2	0.05–0.2	0.15–0.5	900–2700	1525–4575	1400–4200
Adults		70–140	100–200	4–7	2.0–3.0	2.5–5.0	1.5–4.0	0.05–0.2	0.05–0.2	0.15–0.5	1100–3300	1875–5625	1700–5100

a Because there is less information on which to base allowances, these figures are not given in the main table of the RDA and are provided here in the form of ranges of recommended intakes.

b Since the toxic levels for many trace elements may be only several times usual intakes, the upper levels for the trace elements given in this table should not be habitually exceeded.

cium), or by pregnant women (calcium and iron). Others who might need more of a specific vitamin are smokers (vitamin C) and people who don't get outdoors (vitamin D). Specific information on why different people need different amounts of certain vitamins and/or minerals is provided in each of the vitamin and mineral profiles.

The fourth step involves the application of professional judgment. When data are limited or of poor quality, the experts take it upon themselves to interpret what they have and come up with an allowance. If the available data is considered of good quality, no additional interpretation is needed.

Does the RDA Really Mean *Daily?*

The most direct answer to this question is no. The human body is a highly evolved and complex organism with many backup or secondary systems that keep it operating. In the case of vitamins and minerals, the body is able to store excess supplies of these nutrients, in limited quantities, for use on those days when the supplies are short. Thus, the daily needs specified in the RDA do not have to be taken in every day. They can be averaged out over the period of several days or a week without your suffering any adverse effect.

The RDA as a Scientific Standard

The RDA is a standard arrived at by scientists, and nutritionists and others interested in studying human needs of various vitamins and minerals always use it as a guide. The RDA has no legal status, but is used by the federal government when setting the legal standard, known as the U.S. RDA or United States recommended daily allowance.

U.S. RDA

Early attempts by the federal government to regulate the safety and effectiveness of vitamins and minerals in our foods and in supplements resulted in the establishment of a minimal daily requirement (MDR) for six vitamins and four minerals. These were replaced in 1973 when the U.S. Food and Drug Administration published the first U.S. RDA. The U.S. RDA values are derived from the RDA values and are meant to be a simplification of the RDA—to make it easier for manufacturers and food packagers to label their products with nutrient content (see Table 2).

Because the U.S. RDA is promulgated by an arm of the federal government, it carries with it the weight of federal regulation. The U.S. RDA is used as the standard for labeling all consumer products with nutritional value in America, including packaged foods and vitamin supplements.

Information on vitamin and mineral content is always given as "percentage of the U.S. RDA." When calculating your daily vitamin intake from labeled foods, use the actual content, not the percentage listed on the package, since the basis of that percentage may not apply to your age and sex on the RDA table.

Table 2

U.S. Recommended Daily Allowances (U.S. RDA) (For Use in Nutrition Labeling of Foods, Including Foods That Also Are Vitamin and Mineral Supplements)

	Adults and Children Over 4 Years	Infants and Children Under 4 Years
Protein	65 g.*	28 g.*
Vitamin A	5,000 IU	2,500 IU
Vitamin C	60 mg.	40 mg.
Thiamin	1.5 mg.	0.7 mg.
Riboflavin	1.7 mg.	0.8 mg.
Niacin	20 mg.	9.0 mg.
Vitamin D	400 IU	400 IU
Vitamin E	30 IU	10 IU
Vitamin B_6	2.0 mg.	0.7 mg.
Folacin	0.4 mg.	0.2 mg.
Vitamin B_{12}	6 mcg.	3 mcg.
Pantothenic acid	10 mg.	5 mg.

Source: Federal Register 38:20717 (1973).
*If protein efficiency ratio of protein is equal to or better than that of casein, U.S. RDA is 45 g. for adults and 20 g. for infants.

RDA vs. U.S. RDA

The RDA represents the most detailed and logical approach to daily vitamin requirements available to the American public. It is far from perfect and, because individual decisions must be made during the establishment process, is subject to a great deal of comment, criticism, and possible scorn as an unscientific effort. Nevertheless, it is the best we have and has been designated the "gold standard" of *The Vitamin Book* for all of the vitamins and minerals it covers.

The U.S. RDA was rejected as our standard because of the extremely general nature of its listings. It contains only two age classifications (the RDA has ten), does not differentiate between the sexes (the RDA has separate listings for males and females at all ages), and differs from the RDA for at least two vitamins (B_{12} and E).

foreign and International Standards

Some countries simply adopt the FAO/WHO recommendations as their own. In other countries, agencies concerned with nutrition utilize a number of different studies and surveys. Logically, one would think that human nutrient needs are identical for all people, regardless of the country they live in, and that daily requirements should, therefore, be the same for everyone. In fact, the research data on vitamins and minerals is the same, but it is subject to slight differences in interpretation.

Some differences between recommended daily allowances in the United States and Canada and England and FAO/WHO recommendations are given in Table 3.

What If You Take in MORE or LESS Than the RDA for a Vitamin or Mineral?

What happens if you don't take in as much of a given vitamin or mineral as called for by the RDA? What happens if you take in much more than is recommended? Unfortunately, these simple questions require a complicated answer, but here are some important points to remember in considering the RDA for each vitamin and mineral:

1. The RDA value for each nutrient is not an absolute measure of what your daily intake should be. It is only a guide to the amounts of nutrients appropriate for good health; specific needs can vary from one person to the next.

Table 3
Foreign and International Nutrient Standards (Adults)

	United States	Canada	United Kingdom	FAO/WHO
Vitamin				
A	1,000–1,200 mcg.*	800–1000 mcg.	750 mcg.*	750 mcg.
C	60 mg.*	45–60 mg.	30 mg.*	30 mg.
D	5–7.5 mcg.	2.5 mcg.	10 mcg.*	2.5 ug.*
E	12–15 IU*	5–10 mg.	†	†
Biotin	100–300 mcg.	100 mcg.	†	†
Cyanocobolamine (B₁₂)	3 mcg.*	2 mcg.	†	†
Folic acid	0.4 mg.*	0.175–.22 mg.	0.3 mg.*	0.4 mg.*
Nicotinic acid	14–19 mg.*	14 mg.	15–18 mg.*	6.6 mg. 1000 calories
Pantothenic acid	4–7 mg.	5–7 mg.	†	†
Pyridoxine (B₆)	2–2.2 mg.*	1.1–1.8 mg.	†	†
Riboflavin (B₂)	1.2–1.7 mg.*	1 mg.	1.3–1.6 mg.*	1.3–1.8 mg.
Thiamin (B₁)	1.1–1.4 mg.*	0.8 mg.	0.7–1.3 mg.*	0.9–1.3 mg.
Mineral				
Calcium	800 mg.*	700–800 mg.	500 mg.*	†
Iodine	150 mcg.*	160 mcg.	150 mcg.*	**
Iron	10–18 mg.*	7–14 mg.	10–12 mg.*	5–14 mg.*
Magnesium	300–350 mg.*	200–250 mg.	†	300 mg.*
Zinc	15 mg.*	8–9 mg.	†	10 mg.*

*Additional requirements for pregnancy and lactation
†No standard given.
**In 1973, the WHO Expert Group on Trace Elements in Nutrition recommended that high protein food supplements contain 28 mcg. of iodine per 100 calories.
Sources:
Recommended Dietary Allowances. 9th Edition Revised 1980. National Academy of Sciences, Washington DC. 1980; *The Extra Pharmacopeia,* 28th Edition, London, 1982; *Recommended Nutrient Intakes for Canadians.* Minister of National Health and Welfare, Ottawa, Canada. 1983.

2. It is possible to maintain good health even if you don't reach the RDA for some vitamins. Remember, the RDA has been adjusted upward twice, and individual needs will vary considerably.

3. If you are planning to satisfy all of your vitamin and mineral requirements through diet, you will inevitably take in more than the minimum amounts of some vitamins. Not only do foods contain more than one vitamin and/or mineral, the vitamin content of foods is uneven and, in some cases, not completely known.

4. If your regular diet provides more than the RDA of certain nutrients, be careful about the vitamin supplements you use; it is possible to take excessive amounts of some vitamins and minerals.

Each vitamin and mineral must be considered individually when it comes to symptoms of deficiency or the possibility of toxicity. These potential problems are discussed in detail in the individual vitamin and mineral profiles in Parts II and III. However, some generalizations can be made by category.

Water-soluble vitamin deficiencies, except B_{12}, usually make themselves known sooner than those of the fat-soluble vitamins because the body retains much smaller amounts as backup storage. The actual appearance of deficiency symptoms, however, may take a month or more depending on personal circumstances. For example, active people will show deficiency symptoms of the B-complex group involved in body reactions that generate and use energy sooner than sedentary individuals because they are using the vitamins at a more rapid pace.

As a ground rule, most water-soluble vitamins are not toxic, even when you take more than you can possibly use, because the excess is eliminated through the urine. As a result, there tends to be a general lack of concern on the part of most health professionals about severe adverse effects from self-medicating with megadoses of this category of vitamin.

However, as you might expect, there are exceptions, and these are vitamin B_{12}, B_6 and, to some extent, vitamin C. Vitamin B_{12} can accumulate in the body to a toxic level and is stored in the liver and B_6 is also stored in the liver. In the case of vitamin C, the body normally stores in body tissues about 1,500

24

mg. (1.5 g.). After using its daily requirement of ascorbic acid of about 60 mg., the body will ordinarily discard, through the urine, any vitamin C in excess of the 1,500 mg. it already has stored. But when the backup, or inventory, is partially depleted, perhaps because of reduced intake or unusually high use to fight infection, the body will replenish its inventory from either food or vitamin supplements, until the limit of 1,500 mg. has been reached. After that, the body will return to using its 60 mg. a day and discard any additional vitamin C in the urine. Vitamin B_6 has recently been observed to be toxic in doses over 2 grams.

Deficiencies of most fat-soluble vitamins will reveal themselves only after extensive body stores are used up, a process that can take months. On the one hand, this is bad because a diet deficient in these important nutrients is masked for quite a long time and once the deficiency makes itself known through the development of a deficiency disease very large amounts of the vitamin are required to replace the depleted stores and return you to a healthy state. On the other hand, huge stores of fat-soluble vitamins can offer some protection if you find yourself in an unusual circumstance where you are unable to supplement your intake of fat-soluble vitamins.

Fat-soluble vitamin deficiency can be caused by some drugs. For instance, taking the vitamins together with mineral oil—a widely used laxative—because they can dissolve in the mineral oil. If this happens, the vitamins will be eliminated from the body when the mineral oil is eliminated, instead of being emulsified and absorbed into the bloodstream.

Among the fat-soluble vitamins, only relatively amounts of vitamins E and K are stored in the body, even when large doses of these vitamins are taken but they too can be toxic. If you take more vitamin A and D than you need, the excess will accumulate in your liver and body fat, where it will remain. Health professionals are rightly alarmed by people who self-medicate with high doses of A and D because toxicity symptoms can develop from accumulated amounts.

Minerals present somewhat different problems in terms of inadequate or excessive intake. Relatively small amounts of minerals are needed by the average person, and deficiencies in most minerals are therefore rare. The only major exceptions are the high incidence of iron deficiency in women during childbearing years and calcium depletion in the postmenopausal years that may be aggravated by a lifelong calcium deficiency.

Several of the minerals are conveniently stored in large quantities in the form in which they can best serve the body. Calcium, for example, is stored in the structure of bones and teeth; zinc and other minerals are stored as enzyme or protein complexes; magnesium also makes up a part of bones and teeth. This storage potential, though beneficial, can, however, also lead to toxicity. The body's metabolic machinery is not very efficient in rapidly eliminating an excess of an inorganic element like a mineral. Taking as little as two or three times the required amount can be toxic for some minerals. And what makes matters worse is the fact that we don't know the exact amounts of minerals required. For example, copper, which is recommended for adults in daily amounts of 2–3 mg., becomes toxic if it is taken in doses of 10 mg. or more per day. Fluoride is recommended in daily doses of 2.5 mg. to prevent the formation of tooth cavities; however, people taking 10–20 mg. of this element per day can develop a toxic condition in which tooth enamel becomes weakened, discolored, and more susceptible to decay.

Another consideration in determining correct intake is the fact that interaction between vitamins or minerals may impede the absorption of one or both vitamins or minerals. When one is ingested in excess, it may inhibit the availability of one or more other minerals. These interactions take place mainly between minerals with similar electronic structures. They have been discovered in studies on farm animals and in some cases in laboratory animals. The best-known example is the interaction between copper and molybdenum, which was discovered in cattle who develop a disease called scours when grazing on pasture where the herbage contained high levels of molybdenum. The copper deficiency occurred even when copper levels in the plants were considered to be in the normal range. The mechanism by which molybdenum causes a copper deficiency is not well understood, but there appears to be both decreased copper absorption and decreased copper utilization. Some other interactions are listed below, and those considered important to humans are discussed in the respective profiles in Part III.

• Manganese and cobalt interfere with iron.

- Zinc, cadmium, sulfate, and mercury interfere with copper.
- Sulfate interferes with selenium.
- Chromium and vanadium may interfere with each other.
- Phosphorous and zinc interferes with calcium.

The Megadose Issue

People taking massive amounts of some vitamins and minerals to treat conditions unrelated to nutrition, either on their own or as prescribed by a doctor, are using these substances as drugs, not as food supplements. More information on this controversial topic will be found in Chapter 5, "Vitamins and Minerals as Drugs," and in each of the individual vitamin and mineral profiles in Parts II and III.

3

Getting Vitamins and Minerals from the Food You Eat

Most nutrition experts will agree that the foodstuffs of the United States and other industrialized nations have the capacity to provide all the nutrients we need. Yet, many of us are deficient in one or more of these nutrients, or would be if we did not take supplemental vitamins and minerals.

The vitamin inadequacy of the average diet can be verified by information gathered from the most recent national health survey. According to "Caloric and Selected Nutrient Values for Persons 1–74 Years of Age," published by the National Center for Health Statistics, our population is incredibly vitamin deficient. Calcium intake is below acceptable standards in 19 percent of American men and 44 percent of American women. Iron intake is below standard in 45 percent of men and an amazing *82 percent* of women. Vitamin A intake was below standard in almost 44 percent of men and more than 45 percent of women. Thiamin and riboflavin were less of a problem, with intake reported as being below standard in only 6 percent of men and women. If we couple this information with the fact that vitamin deficiencies are more likely to occur in certain groups of people—as discussed in the next chapter—the picture of a society deficient in vitamins and minerals begins to develop.

Why is this? Is modern agriculture destroying the quality of our food? Are our diets inadequate to our needs? Are the RDA's too high? Are we storing and processing our foods improperly? This chapter attempts to shed some light on these important and controversial questions.

Controversy Over Agricultural Methods

Some people are concerned that our soils are becoming depleted of trace minerals by continuous agricultural use and hence that foods are becoming depleted in vital minerals. This is a complex issue about which not a great deal is known, but the lack of evidence of mineral deficiencies in our population speaks to the adequacy of our soil. Furthermore, soils are replenished in trace minerals by rainwater and especially by irrigation water that is obtained from rivers or wells that draw from other soil or rock formations far away from the farm.

On the other hand, agricultural practices that remove the total crop from the field year after year with no replenishment of trace minerals can over time result in a crop poor in these minerals. Of course, the farmer could apply fertilizer to the fields, but with most fertilizers this practice would only replenish potassium, phosphates, and nitrogen. Rotating a "green manure" crop such as clover, which is plowed under after the end of the growing season, would only renew nitrogen in the soil, not trace elements. There is a growing realization, therefore, that so-called organic farming makes good commercial sense and would help minimize mineral depletion. Organic farming essentially means no reliance on chemical fertilizers; rather, soils are invigorated by application of manure and by plowing in crop wastes such as corn stalks and bean vines, and compost. These techniques return organic material and trace minerals back to the soils and are to be commended. However, for maximum yields, a chemical fertilizer may be required in addition to manure and plant waste.

Some critics of modern farming methods fear that the hardier species of fruits and vegetables that have been developed to make shipment easier have resulted in loss of vitamin content.

This concern is unfounded because the creation of vitamins by plants is an automatic biological process. Any variety of plant will make the full complement of vitamins it needs, regardless of species.

On the other side of the fence, several popular writers have advanced the notion that extensive vitamin and mineral supplementation of animals has resulted in excess nutrients finding their way into our diet. In fact, most of the nutrients fed to animals are used up within their own bodies to carry out normal metabolic activities. Any remaining vitamins might be stored as they would in the human body, but otherwise they are simply passed out via the urine.

In our opinion, critics of American agricultural methods—insofar as they reflect on nutrition—have not made a case for their point of view. We must look elsewhere to find out why we do not get all the vitamins and minerals we need from the food we eat.

Can You Eat Enough to Satisfy Your Vitamin and Mineral Needs?

In theory, yes. In practice, probably not.

Surveys have shown that few of us are able to meet the established RDA for all vitamins and minerals through dietary means. We either can't eat the volume of food that would be required to provide the nutrients, don't want the calories found in the foods required to obtain the necessary vitamins because we might gain weight, or simply won't devote the time needed for selecting the proper foods. And many of us won't give up the so-called junk foods that clutter our diets.

In addition, large amounts of some vitamins are lost from foods that have been subjected to the processing techniques normally used in the food industry. These include the treatment of foods prior to canning or freezing, involving sterilization by heat or irradiation, and other processes to which our food is subjected before we actually eat it.

Since it is difficult for most of us to meet normal vitamin and mineral requirements through dietary measures, it follows that achieving higher individual levels of vitamin and mineral intake by dietary means is almost impossible. For example, if you wanted to get an additional 500 mg. of vitamin C from your diet every day, you would have to eat an *extra* 2.5 cantaloupes (400 calories), 7.75 pounds of blueberries (2,200 calories), or 6.5 cups of grapefruit sections (550 calories). You could mix your fruits with other vitamin C sources for variety but would still have to eat an awful lot of extra food. If you wanted an additional 400 units of vitamin E from everyday foods, you would have to eat twenty-one cups of sunflower seeds (17,100 calories), four pounds of English walnuts (11,812 calories), or twenty cups of black raspberries (2,000 calories).

Nutritional needs at higher levels than the RDA are discussed in the individual vitamin and mineral profiles (see Parts II and III), and supplements to daily diet would clearly be needed in such cases. For the average person, some supplements may also be necessary to bring daily intake up to the RDA level, even when serious attention is paid to food intake. Theorists have attempted to work up an ideal "average diet" and nutritionists have set goals for a "balanced diet," but even these have drawbacks when considered in the context of today's lifestyles.

The "Average Diet" Theory

It would be nice, if it were possible, to offer a cookbook solution to the problem of good nutrition by drawing up diets that would be right for everyone. Unfortunately, this is not as easy as it sounds, for several reasons:

First, foods that are commonly found in one area of the country or in one ethnic or economic group may be uncommon in another. There is also wide variation in people's eating habits, even within ethnic groups and regions of the country.

Second, a diet evaluation must include only food that is actually eaten. If considerations are based only on what is bought or prepared, the resulting nutritional picture will be distorted.

Third, the way you prepare and cook raw and processed foods at home may affect their vitamin content. For example, paring certain vegetables before cooking often results in the loss of most of their water-soluble vitamins. Baking and other cooking methods can also lead to vitamin loss.

When estimating the vitamin losses from your food during

preparation, remember that even the smallest quantity of food can be affected. It is unreasonable to expect that the preparation conditions of test foods will be identical to those being prepared in your home. Therefore, individual diets can only be evaluated by analyzing the final food product.

Fourth, your dietary or body level of one vitamin or mineral may influence your requirement for another. For example, many of the water-soluble vitamins' functions are interrelated because they all participate in the series of chemical reactions known as the Krebs cycle, which are involved in energy generation. Thus, a deficiency in one vitamin may affect the ability of other vitamins to function. The nutrients that are interrelated in this way are niacin, thiamin, pyridoxine, riboflavin, biotin, pantothenic acid, choline, and cyanocobalamine.

Vitamin need can also be related to the nature of your dietary intake. Thiamin, niacin, riboflavin, and other water-soluble vitamin requirements are increased in a high carbohydrate diet, while a high protein diet calls for excess pyridoxine and also has an effect on the amount of riboflavin the body stores.

Zinc seems to play a role in the action of vitamin A, so that vitamin A deficiencies can be more easily corrected if there is a sufficient amount of zinc in the diet.

Vitamin C is a factor in the efficient absorption of iron from the gastrointestinal tract. Thus, it is possible that you are taking enough iron but don't have enough ascorbic acid in the diet to get the full value of that iron. Usually, though, the situation is reversed, with more than enough C and too little iron in the diet.

Fifth and last, it is difficult and time-consuming to translate information from nutrition value tables to our daily diet. For example, to determine the vitamin content of a simple ham sandwich on white bread, we must find the listing for: "Ham: piece, approx. 4.125 in. long, 2.25 in. wide, 0.25 in. thick; wt. 1.5 oz."

Assuming that three such slices are used on our sandwich, we can determine that, from the ham alone, we will gain no vitamin A, 7.2 mg. of niacin, 0.37 mg. of riboflavin, 0.81 mg. of thiamin, and no vitamin C. Similar steps must be followed for every part of the sandwich, and then for total food intake.

Interestingly, the technology explosion has led to the introduction of a number of programs and services that will analyze your diet for vitamin and mineral content using a computerized listing of the information contained on the USDA tables entitled "Nutritive Value of American Foods." If such programs become widely available and if people have the time and patience to enter their diet data into their computers, it should be possible to make strides toward the ideal diet. Meanwhile, it remains a theory.

The "Balanced Diet" Goal

Over the years, nutrition and food researchers have developed a set of standard recommendations for the kinds of foods we should eat to maintain a healthy nutritional state. All foods have been very conveniently divided into four categories, each of which provides a portion of our nutritional requirements and should be included in our daily diet.

The Basic Four

I. *Milk Group*
The milk group is typified by whole cow's milk. However, cheese, ice cream, and other foods made from milk can be used to supply the nutrients we would normally get from milk.

II. *Meat Group*
The meat group consists of meats, fish, poultry, and eggs. Dried beans, peas, and nuts may be used as substitutes.

III. *Fruits and Vegetables*
The fruit and vegetable group includes any and all fruits and vegetables.

IV. *Breads and Cereals*
The bread group includes all grains and grain products. Some examples of items from the bread group are rice, cereals, cakes, and of course, all kinds of breads.

Table 4

U.S. Department of Agriculture Food Intake Recommendations

Sample Foods	Serving Size	Servings by Age Group
Milk Group		
		Children (to 9 years): 2–3
Whole milk	1 cup	Children (9–12 years):3
Plain yogurt	1 cup	Teenagers: 4
Ice cream	1½ cups	Pregnant Women: 3
Cottage cheese	2 cups	Nursing Mothers: 4
		Adults: 2–3
Meat Group		All ages: 2
Lean meat	2–3 ounces (cooked)	
Poultry	2–3 ounces	
Fish	2–3 ounces	
Hard cheese	2–3 ounces	
Eggs	2–3	
Cottage cheese	½ cup	
Dried beans and peas	1–1½ cups cooked	
Nuts and seeds	½–¾ cup	
Peanut butter	4 tablespoons	
Fruits and Vegetables		
Cut vegetables	½ cup	All ages: 4
Cut fruits	½ cup	Include at least one good
Grapefruit	½ medium	source of vitamin C, such
Melon	1	as oranges or orange juice,
Potato	1 medium	and one dark green or deep
Salad	1 bowl	yellow vegetable.
Lettuce	1 wedge	
Breads and Cereals		
Bread	1 slice	All ages: 4
Cooked cereal	½–¾ cup	Use whole or enriched
Dry cereal	1 ounce	grains only. Include at least
Pasta	½–¾ cup	1 serving of whole grain.
Rice	½–¾ cup	

The Basic Four, as they have come to be known, were first developed in the 1950s and included recommendations on the amounts of foods to be consumed from each group. Since then these recommendations have undergone a couple of overhauls. The latest was started by Senator George McGovern as chairman of the Senate Select Committee on Nutrition and Human Needs, and in 1977 a new set of nutritional guidelines was published. At that time, the committee recommended a reduction in our intake of cholesterol, fat, salt, refined and processed sugars, alcohol, and calories and an increase in our intake of complex carbohydrates and roughage. These views have been endorsed by the Food and Drug Administration and the U.S. Department of Agriculture.

These changes are not inconsistent with the Basic Four concept. They merely reemphasize which foods should be eaten from which groups. The McGovern Committee goals can be realized by eating more fruits, vegetables, and whole grains, reducing our junk food intake (sweet, fatty, salty, alcoholic), and choosing meats, poultry, fish, and dairy products that are lower in saturated fat and cholesterol.

As an aid to following the Basic Four concept, the U.S. Department of Agriculture has recommended that you eat specified amounts of food from each group as defined on Table 4. Clearly, most people would not fulfill their requirement with one food from any given group. For example, a nursing mother who needs four servings from the milk group every day is not likely to eat eight cups of cottage cheese but might consume the correct amount by having 1 cup of cottage cheese, 2 cups of milk, and 1 cup of plain yogurt.

A typical daily menu designed to meet requirements of a "balanced diet" could look something like this:

Breakfast: ½ cup orange juice
½ cup oatmeal
1 soft-cooked egg
1 cup milk
1 slice toast with butter or margarine

Lunch: 1 cup chicken soup with rice
roast turkey sandwich with mayonnaise
lettuce and tomato with French dressing
1 apple
1 cup coffee or tea

Dinner: 3 ounces broiled veal chop with gravy
½ cup noodles

½ cup coleslaw
½ cup fruit gelatin dessert
1 roll with butter or margarine
coffee, tea, or other beverage

How adequate is this carefully planned menu in meeting our daily vitamin needs? Let's see.

Analysis based on information found in the Vitamin and Mineral Content of Foods tables, beginning on page 307, reveals that, for an adult, this menu is deficient in calcium, vitamin B_6, and folic acid. The level of iron is sufficient for adult males and children between the ages of four and ten. But it has only two-thirds of the iron needed by females between ages eleven and fifty and teenage boys (eleven to eighteen years).

You can determine the vitamin adequacy of your own diet by using the same tables, and it is likely that even if you follow the latest nutritional requirements you could benefit from supplemental vitamins.

Tips on Buying, Storing, Cooking Food

Buying food knowledgeably, storing carefully, and using cooking methods that preserve vitamins and minerals can greatly enhance the nutritional value of the foods in your diet.

Buying

Buy cereals and breads made from whole grains rather than processed grains. Most of the vitamins and minerals are removed in the milling process. Some but not all of those nutrients are replaced if the grain is "enriched." If you can't find whole grain products, try for an enriched (but processed) product. Nonenriched, processed products are the least desirable.

Only use milk products that have been fortified with vitamins A and D. Since the natural vitamin A and D content of milk is lost during homogenization, it must be replaced before you buy the milk. Skim milk and nonfat dry milk products must also be fortified with A and D.

Frozen meats, fish, and poultry are essentially equal to their fresh counterparts when it comes to vitamin and mineral content. Fresh vegetables and fruits may take several days or weeks to reach you, during which time they can begin to lose vitamin content. We believe that fresh vegetables and fruits should be your first choice, but only within a few days of having been picked. The flash-freezing process used to prepare frozen foods does not result in vitamin losses, except for vitamin E. Frozen vegetables that you buy in a plastic cooking pouch are the best kind of frozen product. They maintain their full vitamin content through the cooking process because of the sealed pouch.

Avoid canned vegetables. Any water-soluble vitamins left in the vegetables after processing dissolve in the water used in the packing process and are lost for nutritional purposes.

Fresh fruits are preferable to canned fruits because of potential losses of their water-soluble vitamin content during storage. Frozen fruits will maintain their vitamin content in the same way as frozen vegetables do.

Color may be an indicator of vitamin content. For example, vitamin A is orange in color, and those foods with a high vitamin A content, such as carrots, reflect that color. When buying fresh fruits and vegetables, look for those with a deep, rich color.

Don't keep fresh fruits around the house until they are overripe. The continuing enzymatic process of fruit ripening can lead to the loss of valuable vitamin content. If you buy fresh produce, buy only enough to last a few days (no more than a week).

Homegrown fruits and vegetables are not nutritionally superior to the kind you can buy in your supermarket. However, they usually taste better because they are allowed to ripen before you pick and eat them.

Storing

Make sure your freezer maintains a temperature of 0° F. or less. If the temperature rises above that level, the frozen products may begin to thaw and lose some of their vitamin content. In addition, some frozen products have been found to lose vitamin content after prolonged storage of a year or more, so you should not store them for more than two or three months before use.

Vegetables should be placed in a watertight plastic bag and stored in a refrigerator. Today's frost-free refrigerators are the worst thing for fresh vegetables because they automatically withdraw moisture from the air in the refrigerator. Since water-soluble vitamins will be lost with the moisture extracted from the vegetables, vegetables not stored in watertight plastic bags will lose their vitamin and water content more rapidly than those that are.

Canned foods should not be stored in a very hot environment. The breakdown of vitamins is a chemical process. Like all chemical processes, this breakdown is more rapid when temperatures are higher. Therefore, maintaining your pantry in a cool place will minimize vitamin losses from canned foods.

Store milk and bread away from the sun or strong light, which can destroy their riboflavin content. Clear glass milk bottles should not be used for this reason.

Orange juice will begin to lose vitamin C after it has been stored in your refrigerator for several days, regardless of the container in which it is stored. Don't keep more than you will be able to use in a week's time. Powdered drinks with supplementary vitamin C will hold their vitamin content for a long time and may be an acceptable alternative to fresh or frozen juice products for some people even though they have no other nutrients.

If you pick tomatoes before they are ripe, allow them to ripen in a cool (not cold), dark place. They can be easily ripened by storage in a paper bag. Ripening under any other conditions will result in the loss of some of their nutrients.

Preparing and Cooking

Use the minimum cooking time necessary. High temperatures over short periods of time are preferable to low temperatures over longer periods of time.

The kind of pot used to cook your vegetables or meat does not significantly affect the vitamin content of the final product and may add some of their metal component to your food. Copper, iron, brass, or alloy metals may destroy some vitamin C in the foods being cooked, but the small losses attributed to the pot are unimportant.

Vegetables, including potatoes, retain more vitamins if they are cooked whole than if they are cooked in pieces. The smaller the pieces, the more vitamins lost.

Don't soak fresh vegetables or rice for prolonged periods of time before you cook them. You may soak the water-soluble vitamins right out of them. If you must soak your vegetables, reuse the water.

Prepare salads and cut vegetables just before you intend to eat them. This will reduce the loss of vitamin C.

Do not thaw frozen vegetables before cooking.

Vegetables will lose the most vitamins if boiled, but steaming is not as harmful with respect to vitamin loss. Cooking your vegetables in a pressure cooker is the best way to avoid vitamin losses.

If you do boil fresh vegetables, use minimum amounts of water. When possible, reuse the same water for sauces, gravies, or stock because this water retains many of the vitamins from the vegetables cooked in it.

Meats that are stewed or braised lose more vitamins than those that are fried or broiled. Stewing or braising allows water-soluble and some fat-soluble vitamins to be removed in the gravy. Rare meat has more thiamin, a heat-sensitive vitamin, than meat cooked for longer periods of time.

Precooking foods and storing them in the refrigerator for reheating can result in the loss of a lot of their vitamin C. This is a significant problem for some people because vitamin C is not found in a wide variety of common foods.

If you follow the practices we recommended for cooking foods to minimize vitamin losses, you will also minimize mineral losses. Avoid boiling foods for long periods of time, and use the cooking water as part of your meal. Steaming foods will cook them equally well and minimize nutrient losses.

4

Who Needs Supplemental Vitamins and Minerals?

As discussed in the previous chapter, it may sound reasonable for an average, healthy adult to assume that most of his or her vitamin needs are being met by dietary intake, but this is frequently not so. In particular, this assumption may not be true for *you*. The only way to determine this is by critically examining the nutrients contained in the foods you eat every day.

In addition, you should take into account the fact that at times your normal need for vitamins and minerals is increased. This can happen, for example, during periods of increased body growth, when you are ill, and when you make changes in your diet or exercise program. In reviewing situations that can dictate a need for more vitamins and minerals, this chapter will first talk about age groups and then categories of people that cut across age groups. Finally, it will consider some instances when illness and medication use can affect your vitamin and mineral needs. Table 6 at the end of the chapter summarizes the various circumstances that indicate a need for supplements.

Supplement Needs: Infancy to Old Age

Infants and Young Children

Infants and children under the age of eleven have special vitamin needs. Although children need more vitamins per pound of body weight because of the rapid rate at which they burn energy and use calories, their overall needs for vitamins and minerals are generally lower than those of the adult because they are so much smaller. Notable exceptions to this rule are vitamin D and iron.

Vitamin D plays an important role in the processing of calcium and phosphorous in the body, two major components of bone. Growing infants and children must have enough vitamin D to assure the development of strong bones and teeth.

Iron is a component of the protein called hemoglobin, the function of which is to carry oxygen to body cells. An infant grows at so rapid a pace that it needs much more oxygen per pound of body weight than an adult does. Therefore, it needs as much or more iron than an adult, despite its smaller size. Many pediatricians prefer to give their patients vitamin supplements that contain iron to be sure that they get enough during those critical years.

The RDAs for infants are based on the known content of mother's milk. Since infants thrive when breastfed, setting the RDAs at this level was a natural conclusion. However, an infant who is not breastfed may need supplemental iron and vitamins. These are easily provided in the form of vitamin drops that can be purchased in any pharmacy, both with and without iron. Infants fed commercially prepared formulas do not need supplemental vitamins, including vitamin D and iron (when specified as an ingredient on the bottle or can) because their formulas contain enough extra nutrients to be considered vitamin supplements. The formulas are designed to provide everything the infant will need to grow and thrive.

There is some disagreement among nutritionists about the utility of vitamins and minerals, especially zinc, in commercial formulas versus that in mother's milk. That is, the commercial formulas have more in them because their nutrients are absorbed less efficiently than those obtained from mother's milk. Studies have confirmed the relative differences in absorption, but infants fed by either method will thrive.

Young children can present a more difficult problem than infants because of the food choices they make. Often, children refuse to eat the very foods they need to provide the basic nutrients needed for growth and development. If your child is one of those who refuses to eat properly, a vitamin supplement is advisable. When choosing a vitamin supplement for your child, don't forget to choose one that includes iron, if iron-rich foods are not a part of his or her diet. Dietary surveys continually show iron deficiency to be one of the most frequent problems in all age groups.

Try to vary the foods offered to your child among those that can be particularly good sources of vitamins and minerals. Many vegetables, fruits, grains, and milk products are enjoyed by young children and can serve as the basis for a sound diet.

Teenagers

Teenagers have special vitamin needs because of the tremendous growth spurt they go through and the changes in their bodies induced by sexual maturity and the influence of sex hormones. Boys usually grow by adding muscle and bone. Girls also add muscle and bone, but a larger percentage of their body weight is made up of fat. This, combined with the facts that teenage boys sometimes are more active than girls and that girls have special requirements because of menstruation, sets up some special needs for teenage boys and girls.

Every teenager needs more vitamin D, phosphorous, and calcium than the average adult because of the growth spurt that occurs between the ages of eleven and eighteen years. This need is directly related to the process of building strong bodies and teeth.

Teenage boys need slightly more of the B-complex vitamins than girls. This makes sense when we consider the involvement of B vitamins in our energy-generating system.

Teenage boys and girls need more iron than they did at a younger age, but for different reasons. The need of the teenage girl develops because of the onset of menstruation. Teenage boys need more iron because of their need to supply more oxygen to rapidly growing tissues. Girls will continue to need extra iron until they reach menopause, about age fifty. The iron requirement of the teenage boy goes down by almost 50 percent when growth has stopped and he has passed the teenage years, often signaling a reduction in activity as well.

Teenage girls tend to eat less, sometimes a lot less, than teenage boys. Reducing food intake is fine for maintaining your figure but does nothing to maintain a solid nutritional base. If you assume your teenagers are going to be properly nourished by their diets, you will have to remember that any time food intake is reduced, vitamin and mineral intake is also reduced. We would offer the same suggestion here as for young children. Try to provide a variety of foods that are rich in vitamins and minerals. Fruits, vegetables, and grains are especially good, as are milk and milk products. Supplementary multiple vitamins (with iron) are a good way to ensure that minimum requirements will be met but should not be depended upon as the sole nutrient source for your teenager.

Senior Citizens

Unfortunately, official recommendations for vitamin and mineral intake are subdivided into age groups that end with age fifty. The needs of adults beyond the age of fifty years are grouped into one category: 51 plus.

As you get older, the percentage of fat in your body increases. This fat replaces other tissues (such as muscle), which have a greater need for energy (calories). Because of this change, your basal metabolism, the rate at which the body uses energy, is lowered. To complicate matters, many people tend to engage in less physical activity as they get older, lowering energy requirements even more.

When you reduce both metabolism and physical activity, your need for food energy also decreases. If you were to continue taking in the same number of calories (eat the same amount of food) and use fewer calories each day, your body would store the excess energy as fat. To avoid gaining weight as you get older you eat less food, but when you eat less, you get smaller amounts of vitamins and minerals. Therefore, the need for a general purpose vitamin and mineral supplement increases with advancing age.

Other factors are also present that point to a need for supplemental vitamins and minerals. The bodies of older adults manufacture less of the natural gastrointestinal enzymes and acids needed to digest food, and some older adults cannot chew their food properly. This leads to poor or inefficient digestion and the incomplete extraction of available nutrients from our food.

In addition, many nutritional problems among senior citizens stem from social, economic, and psychological factors. For instance, the loss of close family ties or the illness or death of a spouse can cause depression, which leads to a loss of interest in food and improper nutrition. There are also many older Americans who don't have enough money to buy nutritious foodstuffs.

There have been many studies on the vitamin status of older adults who do not supplement their diets with extra vitamins and minerals. One relatively recent study revealed that 95 percent of senior citizens studied were deficient in at least one nutrient. Ninety percent had low levels of thiamin (vitamin B_1) and vitamin C. When these people were given a B complex with vitamin C supplement, their vitamin status improved and they showed a major improvement in physical and mental condition.

The most reasonable and least costly way for older people to be sure of getting enough vitamins and minerals is to take a well-balanced product with fat- and water-soluble vitamins plus some minerals. Many seniors prefer this solution because it saves them the time and effort of planning and preparing a balanced 2,000-calorie-per-day diet, is economical, and helps prevent overeating of course a well balanced diet is important to obtain adequate nutrients other than vitamins.

Supplement Needs: Special Groups

Pregnant and Breastfeeding Women

Although there is general agreement that pregnant and breastfeeding women need more of every vitamin and mineral, there is no consensus as to specific requirements. This is in spite of the fact that this area of vitamin research has probably been given more attention than any other in recent years.

Vitamin and mineral supplements recommended by the National Academy of Sciences and included in the RDA table are based on the increased energy needs of pregnant women. The NAS estimates that a pregnant woman requires 80,000 *extra* calories during the full term of her pregnancy. Some of these extra calories remain in her body as residual fat stores after the baby is born. All of the extra vitamins and minerals are needed to support the metabolism of these extra 80,000 calories and the growth of her unborn child.

A nursing mother normally produces about 28 ounces of milk each day for a single infant. About one-third of the energy needed to make this milk comes from the extra fat stored during pregnancy. In addition, she may need up to an extra 500 calories per day. In fact, daily energy needs during breastfeeding can actually exceed energy needs during pregnancy.

Studies have shown that pregnant women who are *not* taking vitamin supplements may experience reduced blood levels of vitamins A, B_{12}, and C, nicotinic acid, and pyridoxine. Consequently, the recommendations for increased daily intake of these vitamins during pregnancy and lactation vary between 25 percent and 65 percent above normal adult RDA levels, depending on the vitamin. If you examine listings for virtually all of the vitamins and minerals for which an RDA has been assigned, you will find that pregnancy and lactation are special cases in which the need for extra supplementation has been well documented.

The B vitamins are involved in different phases of the system used to generate energy from glucose (sugar). In fact, many of these vitamins' RDA are based directly on the number of calories we metabolize each day. Thus, it makes sense that during pregnancy, when you use more energy, you need significantly more of the B vitamins to assist in the provision of that energy. It isn't enough to take in the extra calories as food energy, you also have to be able to utilize the energy within the body.

Pregnancy makes great demands on body stores of folic acid. If folic acid stores were low at the beginning of pregnancy because of insufficient dietary intake of the vitamin, there is a good chance that megaloblastic anemia, a disease associated with folic acid deficiency, will develop at some time during the pregnancy.

Vitamin D is also particularly important because it is involved in the formation of strong bones and teeth by helping to mediate the body's use of calcium. Pregnant and breastfeeding women need extra vitamin D to assure proper skeletal development in the unborn child.

These are only a few examples of the need for extra supplies of every vitamin and mineral during pregnancy and lactation. Women who don't take a vitamin supplement especially designed for this period of physical stress are more likely to develop severe vitamin and mineral deficiencies, which can affect the course of their pregnancy, their unborn children, or their general health after the child has been born, since the body will draw many needed nutrients from the mother's body for the baby. Thus, an apparently healthy baby will be born, but the mother may be left in an extremely deficient state. There is evidence to suggest that a vitamin deficient mother may be at a higher risk of giving birth to a child with birth defects.

A note of caution: When selecting a prenatal vitamin, your doctor may prescribe one that he or she has used for years and prescribes out of habit. Many of the formulas meet the RDA for all groups of pregnant women, but some are deficient in the quantity of a vitamin or mineral and others are missing essential nutrients. For example, pregnant women need *at least* 400 international units (10 mcg.) of vitamin D. The RDA for a pregnant woman between the ages of nineteen and twenty-two is 500 units, or 12.5 mcg. This can be easily supplemented by drinking vitamin D–enriched milk or spending some time in the sun, but you should be aware of the potential for deficiency here.

Vitamin E is another problem. Pregnant and lactating women require about 10 mg. (15 international units) of vitamin E each day. Many supplements sold for the specific use of pregnant or lactating women contain no vitamin E. Many others contain sufficient vitamin E. Naturally, you may choose to supplement your vitamin E intake through dietary means.

Calcium is included in vitamin/mineral supplements for pregnant and lactating women, but the amount contained is nowhere near enough to meet your daily requirement. This is especially true of pregnant teenagers, who need 30 percent more than a pregnant adult (1,600 versus 1,200 mg. per day).

Iron is a special problem for pregnant and lactating women of all ages because you can't get enough iron from your diet to meet the special needs of pregnancy and lactation. Your supplemental formula should have between 30 and 60 mg. of iron in it.

For further details on prenatal supplements, see Chapter 6, pp. 78-79.

Pregnant Teenagers

Pregnant teenagers present a special challenge. Although their needs are not significantly different from those of pregnant women, except for the need for even more calcium, a teenager may be less likely to eat foods rich in the nutrients she needs to assure the healthy growth of her baby. Nutritional counseling that stresses the importance of diet and supplemental vitamins and minerals is often helpful in getting the message across to pregnant teenagers.

Athletes

More vitamins are needed when you expend more energy than normal because vitamins are among the raw materials needed for the operation of every cell in the body and the provision of energy to those cells.

Although you cannot expect to improve athletic performance by taking more vitamins than your body can possibly use, as an athlete you should be taking more of the water-soluble vitamins than the inactive person. However, there is no need for excessive vitamin supplementation. Most important are vitamin C, thiamin (vitamin B_1), riboflavin (vitamin B_2) and nicotinic acid (niacin). There are several reasons for this.

First, since athletes tend to be more muscular than nonathletes, your regular energy demands are higher. You need more vitamins to meet these demands since the requirement for so many of these vitamins is directly related to energy expenditure and use of calories. Second, your body metabolism is directly linked to body temperature. Strenuous exercise causes a measurable increase in body temperature and, with it, an increase in the rate of metabolism. When this happens the need for the raw materials of metabolism, including vitamins, also increases. Finally, as you perspire you lose small amounts of all normal body constituents which are ordinarily dissolved in the sweat, including water-soluble vitamins. For the serious athlete, even normal levels of vitamin intake coupled with very high levels of physical activity can therefore result in some vitamin deficiency diseases.

Sweat can also result in loss of excessive amounts of the electrolytes, sodium and potassium. In fact, the problem of electrolyte loss is so great among professional athletes that special replacement solutions containing electrolytes and excess glucose have been developed to permit athletes greater surges of energy and extended periods of athletic activity. The best known of these products is Gator-Ade, but they are not recommended for routine or regular use.

Dieters

The association of vitamin and mineral intake from food with calories is an unavoidable relationship. If, while trying to lose weight, you eat less and exercise more (the *only* way!), the possibility of vitamin deficiency becomes more real than ever. After all, regular exercise only increases your need for some vitamins, as discussed above.

Reducing the number of calories in your daily diet carries with it an automatic reduction in vitamin and mineral intake. This was proven by Dr. Paul LaChance and Michelle Fisher, R.D., of Rutgers University, who evaluated the vitamin and mineral content of ten popular diet plans. The results of their study arc summarized in Table 5. The Pritikin 1200 and F-Diet come the closest to meeting the average person's need, being deficient in two nutrients each. Both provide insufficient levels of vitamin B_{12}; the F-Diet is marginal in calcium, and Pritikin 1200 is marginal in zinc. The Atkins, Beverly Hills, and Richard Simmons diets are the worst, providing adequate levels of only three of the nutrients tested. Stillman and Pritikin 700 follow closely behind, with only four nutrients reaching adequate levels. Clearly, the only way to bridge this obvious gap is to use a vitamin/mineral supplement while dieting or, you might try a more sensible diet.

Vegetarians

Most vegetarians who include animal products in their diets do not need vitamin or mineral supplements, primarily because

Table 5

Nutrient Content of Ten Weight-Loss Diets

Nutrient

Diet	A	C	B₁	B₂	B₃	B₆	B₁₂	Folic Acid	Calcium	Iron	Phosphorous	Zinc	Magnesium
Atkins	M	M	M	M	A	X	A	X	M	X	A	M	X
Beverly Hills	A	A	X	X	X	M	X	A	X	X	X	X	X
F-Diet	A	A	A	A	A	A	X	A	M	A	A	A	A
I Love New York	A	A	X	A	A	M	A	A	M	M	A	M	A
I Love America	A	A	M	A	A	X	X	M	A	M	A	M	M
Pritikin 700	A	A	X	M	M	M	X	A	M	M	A	X	M
Pritikin 1200	A	A	A	A	A	A	X	A	A	A	A	M	A
Richard Simmons	M	A	X	M	A	X	X	X	X	X	A	X	M
Scarsdale	A	A	X	M	A	X	X	M	X	X	M	M	X
Stillman	X	X	X	M	A	X	A	X	X	M	A	A	X

A = Sufficient amounts of this nutrient can be obtained by following this diet.

M = Only marginal amounts of this nutrient can be obtained by following this diet.

X = Insufficient amounts of this nutrient are supplied in this diet. Supplements are needed to maintain daily requirements.

they *are* so conscious of nutrition. Strict vegetarians—or vegans—are, however, very likely to need additional calcium, iron, folic acid and vitamin B_{12}.

Alcoholics

Alcoholics need more of the B vitamins, particularly thiamin, because the alcohol decreases thiamin and folate absorption and utilization into the body. Another important reason for vitamin and mineral deficiency among alcoholics, both recognized and unrecognized, is the fact that alcohol often replaces solid food at mealtimes. This leads to obvious dietary deficiencies of all essential nutrients. While supplemental vitamins and minerals won't cure an alcoholic or allow him or her to go on without worrying about the dire consequences of alcohol abuse, they may be able to replace some of the nutrients missed from a daily diet.

Smokers

Smokers have been shown to use more vitamin C than nonsmokers. This has been verified by studies showing that the usual concentrations of vitamin C in the blood of smokers were lower than those of nonsmokers. This difference was maintained even after vitamin C injections were given to both groups. Some experts have estimated that each cigarette burns 25 mg. of vitamin C and that heavy smokers can lose as much as 50 mg. per day of that vitamin.

Supplement Needs Relating to Medical Problems

Difficulties in Absorbing Vitamins and Minerals

Some people may not be able to absorb vitamins and minerals from their food or from supplemental sources as efficiently as others. The most common causes of this problem are intestinal inflammations such as colitis, bile duct blockage (affects only the fat-soluble vitamins), cystic fibrosis, diarrhea, and aging.

If you have one of these problems you may gain from vitamin supplements because the more vitamin presented to the gastrointestinal tract, the more you are likely to absorb into the blood. The possible benefit offered by vitamin supplements will not be as great, however, if you have permanent absorption problems than it would be if the problem were temporary, as, for instance, diarrhea.

Injury, Severe Burns, Trauma, Surgery, Infection

Each of these situations involves a set of circumstances in which the body is stressed and attempting to heal itself. The healing process requires intense activity on the part of all body systems, especially those involved with the provision of energy and growth of body tissues. Since the vitamins and minerals are integrally involved in these processes, it is logical to assume that vitamin and mineral supplementation will be helpful. In fact, physicians treating hospitalized patients recovering from surgery, severe burns, prolonged infections, and other extended illnesses have long known that nutritional supplementation is one of the basic keys to successful recovery.

Interestingly, many patients have been fed intravenously with mixtures of glucose, amino acids, vitamins, trace minerals, and fats. This technique, known as total parenteral nutrition (TPN), or hyperalimentation, has been used as a temporary supplement in people who can tolerate only small amounts of food and as the sole source of nutrition for people recovering from major surgery, burns, etc. Whereas vitamins have always played a major role in TPN formulas, trace minerals have gained popularity only within the past few years because of recognition of the need to provide small amounts of these elements to people depending on TPN as their sole nutritional source.

Disease

Generations of mothers have known instinctively that good nutrition not only prevents illness but promotes a more rapid recovery from any disease. The better we eat, the faster we get over whatever is ailing us.

Recent research has shown that your mother really did know best. Any stressful situation increases the rate at which your body uses vitamins. Since disease is one form of stress to which the body is exposed, it makes sense to use a vitamin supplement whenever a disease or other physically stressful situation presents itself.

It is also known that deficiencies in vitamin A or C are most likely to make you more susceptible to such ailments as the common cold. With less vitamins, your body is less able to carry out those functions which protect against invading viruses. Taking at least the RDA for both of these vitamins can help speed recovery if you are stricken with a bacteria or virus.

Drug Therapy and Vitamins

There are many instances in which drugs can affect the action of vitamins and in which vitamins can affect the action of drugs when both are present in the body. Here are some of the ways a drug can affect a vitamin:

A drug can interfere with the chemical action of a vitamin. One example is the effect of chloramphenicol, an antibiotic, on folic acid, one of the B-complex vitamins.

A drug can interfere with vitamins being absorbed into the bloodstream from the stomach or intestine. An example of this is the effect of neomycin, an antibiotic, on vitamin B_{12}.

A drug can increase the amount of vitamin absorbed. An example of this is the effect of colchicine, a drug used to treat gout, on vitamin B_{12}.

Some drugs can lead to vitamin deficiency. One example is the effect of hydralazine, a drug used for high blood pressure, on pyridoxine (vitamin B_6).

A drug can increase the rate at which a vitamin is eliminated from the body. An example of this is the effect of phenytoin, a drug used to treat epilepsy, on vitamin D.

Vitamins can affect drugs in the body in several different ways:

A vitamin can counteract or inhibit the effect of a drug. The best example is the effect of vitamin K on the oral anticoagulant (blood-thinning) drugs. Vitamin K is used as an antidote to the effects of the oral anticoagulants.

Vitamins can influence the absorption of drugs through their own effects on body processes. Examples of this situation are the effect of vitamin C on oral iron supplements and the effect of pyridoxine (vitamin B_6) on 1-dopa, used to treat Parkinson's disease. Vitamin C increases the absorption of iron, and B_6 increases the rate at which 1-dopa is broken down.

Very large doses of vitamin C can affect the acidity of the urine and, therefore, affect the urinary elimination of drugs that require a steady level of acidity.

Vitamins can also affect a number of diagnostic tests. For example, large doses of vitamin C can affect certain blood tests for diabetes. Vitamin D can interfere with tests for blood cholesterol levels and other blood tests.

A complete table of known interactions and influences of vitamins on drugs and laboratory tests can be found in Part IV, "Vitamin, Mineral, and Drug Interactions." In addition, each vitamin and mineral profile includes a discussion of such problems, if present.

Table 6
Who Needs Supplements?

People whose vitamin/mineral intake is inadequate due to:
 Dieting
 Heavy alcohol use
 Economic disadvantage
 Old age

People who have extra vitamin/mineral needs:
 Infants
 Young children
 Teenaged boys and girls
 Pregnant women
 Breastfeeding women
 Pregnant teenagers
 Smokers
 Some vegetarians
 People undergoing major surgery
 People subject to severe injury and trauma
 People suffering from disease or prolonged infection

People who have difficulty absorbing vitamins due to:
 Bile duct blockage
 Chronic diarrhea
 Chronic disorders of the stomach and intestine
 Effects of aging

People who are taking drugs that interfere with vitamins
 (See Part IV, "Vitamin, Mineral, and Drug Interactions.")

5

Vitamins and Minerals as Drugs

Even though professional health care is relatively available to most Americans, many of us still use self-help remedies and treatments. This is partly a result of the ever increasing costs of health care and partly due to the reemerging American determination to "do it ourselves." Vitamins and minerals play an incredibly popular role in this social and psychological health care phenomenon.

It is generally recognized by health authorities that doses between three and five times the average adult RDA may be required from time to time for the correction of a vitamin deficiency symptom, when someone has a chronic illness that limits nutritional intake or places a great demand on vitamin use, or when someone is not eating properly. However, when you begin to take vitamins or minerals to treat a condition not related to vitamin deficiency, you have stepped into different territory. Now, you are taking a vitamin or mineral for its effect as a drug.

When used as drugs, vitamins and minerals are frequently taken in large or "mega" doses. A megadose is generally defined as a dose of a nutrient ten or more times greater than the average adult RDA. If no RDA has been assigned, then the megadose is considered to be ten times the U.S. RDA, or the established safe and adequate daily intake. Admittedly, this definition is somewhat arbitrary and some people may suffer vitamin side effects at doses below this, "mega," level, but it serves as a guide for vitamin enthusiasts and critics alike. It may be difficult to exclude vitamin doses that are seven or eight times the RDA from megavitamin discussions, but it is important to establish the megavitamin concept in your mind.

Before taking vitamins as drugs, every consumer must consider both the safety and efficacy of such a program. Since all vitamins are chemicals affecting the body, taking them in excessive doses may cause the system to become overloaded; if that happens, vitamins may yield harmful effects which can far overshadow any possible benefits.

Proponents of vitamin therapy for nondeficiency diseases invariably base their claims on surveys and studies of some sort, but many of these guidelines are, in our opinion, not valid. When we evaluated studies for inclusion in this book, several important criteria had to be met before the study and its conclusions could be considered valid.

• Each study had to demonstrate clearly that the response could be traced to the vitamin under consideration.
• Sampling methods and other experimental procedures had to meet established scientific criteria.
• The methods of analysis had to be appropriate for the particular study method and the information collected.

Outstanding examples of how the facts can be misinterpreted *and* misrepresented may be found in each vitamin and mineral profile in Parts II and III under the heading "Unsubstantiated Claims." These sections include therapeutic uses that have not yet met the rigorous requirements of scientific testing and confirmation. Table 7, at the end of this chapter, also provides a summary of current scientific knowledge about the therapeutic uses of vitamins and minerals. In some cases, such as those of vitamin E and sexual performance, vitamin E as a treatment for muscular dystrophy, and vitamin C as a cancer cure, false claims have led millions of unwary Americans into using vitamins when none was needed or could have helped.

How Facts Can Become Twisted

People who advance unproven theories of vitamin cure for the ills of mankind very often use faulty reasoning in drawing their conclusions. We will briefly review the most common kinds of errors made and illustrate them with some of the most popular vitamin therapies. There is always more than one error associated with each vitamin use, but we will focus on one error in each of the following discussions. More complete information may be found in each of the vitamin and mineral profiles.

Using Anecdotal Reports: Vitamin C and the Common Cold

This kind of faulty reasoning is based on taking the unverified and scientifically uncontrolled experience of one group of people and trying to apply it to everyone. In the case of megavitamins, the uncontrolled experience of thousands or even hundreds of thousands may be taken to draw generalized conclusions.

Vitamin C (ascorbic acid) has been widely promoted as a treatment for the common cold (see page for a detailed discussion). Reports in health and other popular magazines recommend vitamin C doses anywhere from 1,000 mg. to megadoses of 10,000 mg. (10 g.) per day. Unfortunately, the more vitamin C you take, the more likely you are to experience side effects— even though rare—just as you would with any other drug.

Most of the current popularity of vitamin C can be traced to Dr. Linus Pauling, whose claims are based on his personal experiences with early studies on the common cold. These early studies have been criticized by many scientists, who claim their scope and design were not broad enough to support the very general conclusion drawn, that is, that vitamin C will prevent and treat the common cold.

Actually, the effect of vitamin C on the common cold had been studied for many years before it caught Dr. Pauling's eye. As early as 1942, a clinical study did indeed report that students receiving 200 mg. per day of vitamin C had one-third fewer colds. And in 1961, another study done on schoolchildren receiving 1,000 mg. (1 g.) of vitamin C daily showed they also had a third fewer colds. But one recent tabulation of reports and studies published since 1970 indicates that, in over 7,000 subjects tested, the use of vitamin C to prevent or treat the common cold did not show any major benefit. Most results seemed to depend on subjective factors such as age, sex, occupation, and exposure to others ill with colds, flu, and so on.

Attempts scientifically at verifying the value of vitamin C treatment for the common cold have not proven fruitful, and when some positive results have been obtained, they cannot be reproduced by other investigators and are considered invalid.

Using Unverified Reports: Nicotinic Acid (Niacin) and Mental Illness

The practice of treating mental illness with vitamins has been termed orthomolecular psychiatry. Orthomolecular practitioners often quote unverified reports and unreproducible results as the basis for their treatment. Generally, orthomolecular therapy, which has been officially disapproved by the American Psychiatric Association, involves the use of large doses of nicotinic acid plus combinations of the B-complex vitamins and vitamin E.

Many vitamin enthusiasts suggest that mental illnesses— including schizophrenia, which seems to have become the focus of many—will respond to treatment with megadoses of some vitamins. Other claims for vitamin therapy having to do with mental health involve the treatment of depression, anxiety, and stress-related illnesses.

It is interesting to note, however, that psychiatrists and analysts who prescribe megavitamin therapy almost always use other, more conventional forms of therapy (tranquilizers, psychotherapy, etc.) along with the vitamins. This obviously clouds the issue and makes it much more difficult to evaluate the effect of vitamin therapy.

Scientific evaluation of nicotinic acid as a treatment for schizophrenia concludes that improvements claimed by purveyors of the megavitamin therapies resulted not from the vitamins but from the conventional therapy (drugs and/or psychotherapy) given at the same time.

It may also be that some patients are being misdiagnosed as schizophrenics when they are actually manic depressives, a condition in which people exhibit bizarre and uncontrollable behavior while in a severe depression. The mineral lithium is the most effective and important agent used in the treatment of manic depression. Manic depressives being treated with products containing both nicotinic acid and lithium (even in the small amounts in which lithium can be found as a contaminant of the vitamin formula) may be experiencing benefit from the lithium alone.

Ignoring the Placebo Effect: Stress Formula Vitamins

Placebos, or inactive drug products, are often given to patients to soothe and comfort them or to meet a patient's desires. When this occurs, people will show an improvement simply because they are taking something. Sometimes, people complaining of vague and nonspecific symptoms or those who are sad and depressed will show some improvement if given an inactive substance simply because they have been told they will get better. The placebo effect can account for 15–20 percent of the positive response to pain relievers and psychoactive drugs.

When applied to vitamin therapy, the placebo effect can be illustrated by the stress formula products. All of these products contain three to five times the average adult RDA of the B-complex vitamins and ascorbic acid, and some have added vitamin E and minerals. They have been widely promoted as having a positive effect on relieving the symptoms of stress, and in some cases they may have done just that—but *not* because they are vitamins and/or minerals.

The use of vitamins to relieve stress, other than that associated with marginal vitamin deficiency, is simply not reasonable. High doses of vitamins do not have a tranquilizing effect on the central nervous system.

Nevertheless, many manufacturers of multiple vitamin products have developed a "stress formula," which might be represented by the following typical example:

Vitamin	Dose	Percent of Adult RDA
Ascorbic acid	600 mg.	1,000
Thiamin	10 mg.	850
Riboflavin	10 mg.	700
Nicotinic acid (Niacin)	100 mg.	650
Pyridoxine	5 mg.	225
Vitamin B_{12}	15 mg.	500
Pantothenic acid	20 mg.	200*
Vitamin E	30 mg. (45 IU)	225

*There is no RDA for pantothenic acid. The U.S. RDA for adults is 10 mg.

The rationale for this formula is the fact that someone under stress is experiencing a series of physical changes. If we are stressed, we are not eating properly, getting enough sleep or exercise, or leading our normal life. This special combination of vitamins is supposed to substitute for our shortcomings in the stressful situation, despite the fact that reason tells us we cannot continually push ourselves beyond reasonable physical limits without suffering some adverse consequences.

One interesting argument that megavitamin proponents often use is the fact that surgical patients and those undergoing stressful treatments in a hospital are often given nutritional supplements that contain vitamins. It is acknowledged that these patients do better when they have been nutritionally supported, but it is unreasonable to draw the conclusion that the same vitamins which help a surgical patient to heal more quickly will help relieve your daily stresses. In the first case, the vitamins are contributing to the reconstruction and healing of tissues, and in the second they are being taken to help reconstitute a stressed and worn psyche.

Since there have been no conclusive reports to substantiate the stress formula theory, we suggest that stress management be accomplished only under the guidance of qualified medical personnel and not with self-help megavitamins.

Misapplying Animal Data to People: Vitamin E and Chromium

The claim that vitamin E increases human sexual function was based on the observation that rats deficient in vitamin E had reproductive problems. When the rats were given supplemental vitamin E, they were able to reproduce normally.

Vitamin E will not help your sex life, unless you're a rat. Human studies have shown that megadoses of vitamin E in the range of 400–800 units per day can, in some instances, cause side effects that include stomach upset, diarrhea, dizziness, bleeding in people taking oral anticoagulant drugs and *reduced* gonad function. That's right folks, those megadoses of vitamin E can do exactly the opposite of what you are hoping for.

Another example of the improper application of animal studies to humans is the promotion of chromium, an essential mineral, as an aging preventive. Animals in which a chromium deficiency was artificially produced had difficulty metabolizing glucose, fats, and protein. They grew less and died at younger ages than their counterparts given chromium in the diet. This data has led vitamin and mineral enthusiasts to claim that chromium supplements can prevent people from aging. Chromium, in the form of a complex with protein, does play a role in metabolizing glucose, but there is nothing to suggest that supplemental chromium pills can keep you young.

Side Effects from Vitamin/Mineral Overdose

Many people take megadoses of vitamins and minerals without truly understanding the potential problems associated with them. The possible side effects of megadose therapy with vitamins and minerals are discussed in each of the vitamin and mineral profiles. Some of these nutrients, such as vitamin A, vitamin D, thiamin, pyridoxine, folic acid, calcium, phosphorous, chloride, magnesium, potassium, sodium, iron, copper, zinc, fluorine, manganese, and molybdenum, can be toxic when taken in megadoses. Extreme caution must be exercised when considering megadose therapy, especially when the minerals are involved. You should not take large or megadoses of vitamins unless prescribed by your doctor to treat a specific problem or unless a therapeutic use has been scientifically substantiated. The fact that the press or a public figure has publicized the use of one vitamin or another does not make it effective therapy or protect you from possible harmful side effects.

Table 7
Therapeutic Effectiveness of Vitamins and Minerals

Vitamin/ Mineral	Suggested Major Uses	Effec- tive	Slightly Benefi- cial	Not Effec- tive	Infor- mation Lacking
Water-Soluble Vitamins					
Vitamin B₁ (thiamin)	Beriberi prevention and treatment	x			
	Learning disabilities due to "inborn errors of metabolism"	x			
	Nerve tonic			x	
	Insect repellant			x	
Vitamin B₂ (riboflavin)	Conjunctivitis ("red eye")			x	
	Skin diseases			x	
Vitamin B₃ (nicotinic acid)	Pellagra	x			
	High cholesterol	x			
	Heart diseases			x	
	Mental illness/ schizophrenia			x	
Vitamin B₅ (pantothenic acid)	Relief of itching/ soothing of wounds	x			
	Healing of wounds			x	
	Stress			x	
	Graying of hair			x	
Vitamin B₆ (pyridoxine)	Depression due to oral contraceptives	x			
	Learning disabilities due to "inborn errors of metabolism"	x			
	Carpal tunnel defect		x		
	Reduction of breast milk				x
	Morning sickness				x
	Premenstrual syndrome				x

Therapeutic Effectiveness of Vitamins and Minerals

Vitamin/ Mineral	Suggested Major Uses	Effective	Slightly Beneficial	Not Effective	Information Lacking
Vitamin B$_{12}$ (cobolamine)	Pernicious anemia	x			
	Tiredness			x	
Folic acid	Megaloblastic anemia	x			
	Changes in cervical cells and anemia resulting from drop in folic acid level due to oral contraceptives				x
Vitamin C (ascorbic acid)	Scurvy	x			
	Healing of wounds	x			
	Herpes cold sores	x			
	Cold symptoms		x		
	Prevention of colds			x	
	Prevention of infection			x	
	Genital herpes			x	
	Periodontal disease			x	
	High cholesterol			x	
	Cancer				x
	Mental illness				x
	Alcoholism				x
	Drug abuse				x
	Rectal polyps				x
	Bedsores				x
Fat-Soluble Vitamins					
Vitamin A (and retinoic acid)	Cancer	x			
	Acne	x			
	Psoriasis	x			
Vitamin D	Rickets	x			
	Osteomalacia	x			
	Malfunctioning parathyroid gland	x			
	Franconi syndrome	x			
Vitamin E	Cystic breast disease	x			
	Intermittent severe leg muscle pains	x			

Therapeutic Effectiveness of Vitamins and Minerals

Vitamin/ Mineral	Suggested Major Uses	Effective	Slightly Beneficial	Not Effective	Information Lacking
	Nighttime leg cramps	x			
	Healing of wounds		x		
	Protection of the body from the effects of oxygen				x
	Sexual function			x	
	Heart disease/angina			x	
	Athletic performance			x	
	Scars			x	
	Cardiac problems due to chemotherapy				x
	Hemolytic anemia due to G6–PD enzyme deficiency				x
	Enzyme glutathione synthetase deficiency				x
	Environmental hazards such as lead poisoning				x
Vitamin K	Prevention of bleeding in newborn infants	x			
	Antidote to oral anticoagulants	x			
Pseudovitamins					
Choline	Alzheimer's disease		x		
	Liver damage due to alcoholism			x	
	High cholesterol			x	
Inositol	High cholesterol			x	
	Arteriosclerosis			x	
	Stroke			x	
	Heart disease			x	
	Cirrhosis			x	
	Dizziness			x	
PABA	Sunscreen	x			
Laetrile (vitamin B$_{17}$)	Cancer			x	
Essential fatty acids (vitamin F)	Intravenous feeding	x			

Therapeutic Effectiveness of Vitamins and Minerals

Vitamin/ Mineral	Suggested Major Uses	Effec- tive	Slightly Benefi- cial	Not Effec- tive	Infor- mation Lacking
Bioflavinoids (vitamin P)	Bleeding			x	
	Cold symptoms			x	
	Prevention of colds			x	
Essential Minerals					
Calcium	Rickets	x			
	Osteomalacia	x			
	Postmenopausal osteoporosis	x			
	Hypertension				x
Phosphorous	Laxative	x			
Magnesium	Laxative	x			
	Seizures due to toxemia of pregnancy	x			
Iodine	Underactive thyroid and goiter	x			
Iron	Hypochromic microcytic anemia	x			
Zinc	Healing of burns	x			
	Healing of wounds and broken bones	x			
	Arthritis			x	
	Cancer			x	
Important Trace Minerals					
Copper	Heart disease			x	
	Arthritis				x
Manganese	Prevention of aging			x	
Fluoride	Dental caries	x			
	Postmenopausal osteoporosis				x
Chromium	Maturity-onset diabetes	x			
Selenium	Cancer				x
	Prevention of aging			x	

6

How to Buy and Take Vitamin and Mineral Products

As you face shelves filled with vitamin-mineral products, it will soon become obvious to you that formulas vary widely (although there may be more than one company making identical formulas), that there are a variety of different claims made for each formula, and that the terminology used by vitamin manufacturers is not standardized and, therefore, varies tremendously among vendors.

The final decision as to whether you should take a supplement and, if so, what product to take must include consideration of your personal habits, physical condition, eating habits, and medicines you are taking. Most people will do quite well with a regular multivitamin or multivitamin with minerals. The real need for therapeutic formulas, stress formulas, or other special formulas guaranteed to cure what ails you is questionable. The decision to take vitamin products which supply more than 100 percent of the RDA should be made in concert with your doctor or another knowledgeable individual.

Where to Get Advice on Your Vitamin Needs

The first health professional to consider is your family doctor. Many medical schools now teach the basics of nutrition. But most physicians in current practice, like other health professionals, have received virtually no training in the nutrition sciences during their education. Their background in this field has been gleaned from readings in the medical literature, personal experience, and exposure to nutritionists and other physicians who have extensively studied the subject. The best that the average doctor can offer in this area is extensive background and training in disease and its treatment, a knowledge of where to find nutritional information, and good common sense. When asked to recommend a vitamin or vitamin-mineral combination, many physicians will simply recommend that brand of vitamins which they take, other patients have taken, or was the subject of a recent medical advertisement or salesman's pitch. Fortunately, that recommendation is usually as good as any other, and virtually all physicians will recommend vitamin or vitamin-mineral supplements for patients they feel are malnourished or need extra nutritional support.

Some physicians, though, are more nutritionally oriented than others and may, therefore, be more able to recommend a vitamin regimen suited to your individual needs. For instance, most obstetricians and gynecologists will recommend a vitamin-mineral supplement suited for pregnant or breastfeeding women. Sports medicine specialists may recommend a variety of vitamins and minerals for their athlete patients.

Other health professionals can offer solid advice about the role of nutrition and vitamins to specific body functions. For example, your dentist is probably the only person who closely examines your mouth. In doing so, he or she may come upon a sign of vitamin deficiency (B_1, B_2, B_{12}) or a drug side effect. Don't exclude your dentist from discussions relating to nutritional matters; he may have some interesting information to offer.

Your pharmacist is the most accessible and lowest-cost source of health care information and advice. When it comes to vitamin products, most pharmacists are more than willing to include their consultation in the purchase price of the bottle of vitamins. Pharmacists are also exposed to only a minimum of nutritional information during their professional education, and those who have become expert in this field have done so only through information obtained after graduation by taking special courses. While many pharmacists have made the effort to do this, others have not. This means that you must choose your pharmacist as carefully as you would your doctor. A pharmacist who charges you a few pennies more for your prescription or vitamins may be worth it in the long run because of the extra time he takes to be sure that his professional expertise is always up to date.

Nurses, dieticians, and public health counselors are also good information sources when it comes to nutritional matters, although only the dietician has extensively studied nutrition. The problem with these people is that they are usually salaried employees of a hospital or clinic and offer their services only to patients of those facilities. Many registered dieticians have gone into private practice as nutritional counselors. They, and others, specializing in nutrition therapy can be found in the Yellow Pages under "Nutritionists." Look for a person with some professional credentials.

Last, but certainly not least, we cannot forget the thousands of people who own, operate, and work in health food stores or vitamin centers. Many health food people provide common sense information about balanced diets, proper nutrition, and vitamin use, but too many of them feel that vitamins are the cure-all for our daily problems, from the common cold to cancer. If the medical establishment (including the pharmaceutical industry) had the answers to these illnesses, they would have been making and selling them long ago, at a substantial profit. Unfortunately, the answers to so many of the questions that plague us are not known to anyone, including the "vitamin jockeys." Be extremely cautious when someone tells you about vitamins to save or replace your hair or perform some other equally miraculous feat, the miracles of natural (versus synthetic) vitamins, or the aphrodisiac powers of this pollen or that vitamin. These statements are simply untrue and should be considered a form of modern medical quackery.

We are not saying that everything you hear in a health food or vitamin store should be ignored and that everything you hear in a pharmacy should be taken as the gospel. We are simply suggesting that you take everything you hear, regardless of the source, as information to be verified and then acted on. Beware of instant cures and miracles.

One final point. Health food and vitamin stores are in existence because there is a tremendous ($2 billion per year) market for the products they sell. Many pharmacies have dramatically expanded their vitamin centers for the same reason: profit. We don't want to suggest that the sole motive of these people is to sell you as much as they can without regard to your needs. But the fact remains that if they don't sell you something, they can't stay in business.

Understanding Vitamin and Mineral Terminology

When shopping for a vitamin formula, remember that the people who make and market these products use the same techniques to sell them as they use to sell detergents, food products, toothpaste, and other consumer goods.

Market surveys conducted among vitamin and other health product purchasers have shown a strong preference for products that are labeled with the words *natural, high potency, complete formula, super,* or other terms that convey a sense of strength or a link with "natural goodness." Since these words do not have a specific meaning, they can be used in whatever context the manufacturer wishes. Some products give the impression of being high potency but are really the same as regular multivitamins or multivitamins with minerals. Other products are given names that would imply that they are stress or therapeutic formulas but do not fit the profile for these products.

The only way we can suggest to deal with these marketing practices is to ignore them and follow these simple steps:

• Decide what kind of a vitamin you want to take (multivitamin with or without minerals, prenatal formula, etc.).
• Compare labels, on which the content of each vitamin must

be expressed as milligrams and percentage of the U.S. RDA, as well as price.

• Avoid products with gimmicky names, claims, or ingredients.

• Buy the product that meets your need at the lowest price.

How Vitamins Are Measured

One of the things many people find confusing about buying vitamins are the units used to measure them. Most vitamins and minerals are measured in terms of how much they weigh, and since vitamins and minerals are usually needed only in very small quantities, the units of weight of each are very small.

The largest unit of weight you will come across in this book is a gram. One gram is equivalent to about one-fifth of a teaspoon. The abbreviation for gram is "g."

Most vitamins and minerals are measured in milligrams. One milligram is equal to one-thousandth of a gram. The abbreviation for milligram is "mg." However, some vitamins are needed in such small quantities that they are measured in units equal to one-thousandth of a milligram, or one-millionth part of a gram. This unit is called a microgram, and its abbreviation is "mcg." or "ug."

Until 1980, vitamins A, D, and E were officially measured in terms of "international units" or IU, based on measures of biological activity rather than weight. This designation has recently been converted to a weight equivalent to provide more standardization, although you will still see vitamin products labeled in IU because the nomenclature is older and more familiar to most people. The equivalents are:

Vitamin A (retinol)*:   5 IU = 1 mcg.
Vitamin D (cholecalciferol)†:   400 IU = 10 mcg.
Vitamin E: 15 IU = 10 mg.

*All substances with vitamin A activity are included here. Their vitamin activity is expressed in terms of retinol equivalents, one form of vitamin A.

†All substances with vitamin D-like activity are included here. Their vitamin activity is expressed in terms of cholecalciferol equivalents, one form of vitamin D.

Natural vs. Synthetic Vitamins

A major decision faced by the vitamin consumer is whether to buy a ''natural'' or ''synthetic'' (unnatural?) product.

Time and time again, one hears claims that vitamins from ''natural'' sources such as plants or other materials found in nature are actually of higher quality, more effective, and better for you than those manufactured in the laboratory. This is simply untrue.

Since vitamins are identifiable chemicals, the source of the chemical is not nearly as important as the purity and quality of the chemical in determining whether it will be able to do its job. Although the words *natural* and *organic* are in vogue, the only important difference between natural and synthetic vitamins is cost. Natural vitamins must be extracted from plants and involve a complicated, often costly, process. These costs are passed on directly to you in the form of a higher purchase price.

Chelated Minerals

A claim made by some vendors of multivitamin-mineral products is that chelated minerals, that is, minerals attached to an amino acid, are more rapidly absorbed into the system than nonchelated minerals. Some have gone so far as to say that products with minerals that are not chelated to amino acids are the same as those with no mineral content at all. While this may sound reasonable, there is, in fact, no scientific evidence to support such a claim. The only proven value of chelated mineral products is their ability to separate the purchaser from more dollars than the purchaser of traditional vitamin-mineral formulas.

Single Vitamins vs. Multivitamin Products

Is it better to take an all-inclusive product or to determine your individual needs and take each component as a separate pill? Ideally, one might suspect that it would be best to determine *exact* vitamin and mineral needs and then buy each ingredient as a separate product.

While there is nothing wrong with this approach, it is not

the easiest way to be sure of meeting minimal nutritional requirements. Therefore, we recommend that individual supplements be used only when they are specifically indicated. Possible reasons for individual vitamin supplements may be found in the individual vitamin and mineral profiles. If you do decide to buy each vitamin as a separate product, you need not worry about vitamins or minerals interfering with each other; they can be taken together.

Choosing a Multivitamin Product

There are several hundred different brands of multivitamin combinations from which to choose. The major types are described here, and the vitamin and mineral content of the most popular brands are listed in Table 8 at the end of this chapter.

General Multivitamins

Multivitamin formulas contain ten or eleven vitamins, no minerals, and meet most people's vitamin needs. Included in these formulas are vitamins A, C, D, E, thiamin, riboflavin, pyridoxine, and nicotinic acid (niacin) in amounts that approximate the RDA for each of these nutrients. Some multivitamins contain other ingredients such as B_{12}, calcium pantothenate, and even folic acid, but quantities are always in the RDA range. If you choose a formula with folic acid, you will be sure to meet your RDA for all vitamins for which there is an RDA.

General multivitamin combinations are usually among the least expensive of all vitamin products. Some brands are Dayelets, Hexavitamins, One-A-Day tablets, Flintstones, Pals, Unicap tablets or capsules, Vigram tablets, and Zymacap capsules. There are also many generic multivitamin brands available at a substantial savings over some of the brands mentioned. Availability may vary from one area of the country to another so check with your pharmacist or vitamin store for low-cost equivalent products. A word of caution, however: generic multivitamins are not suitable as prenatal supplements or vitamins for breastfeeding women.

Multivitamins with Minerals

These formulas contain both vitamin and mineral ingredients. The quantity of each ingredient needs to be close to the

RDA, where one has been established, although once again it is virtually impossible to classify the specific ingredients of products in this group. Multivitamins with mineral products are promoted as general purpose nutritional supplements. The sales pitch here is simply, ''As long as you're taking a multivitamin, why not take some minerals too. After all, it's just as easy to take a multivitamin mineral product as it is to swallow a vitamin.'' The need for daily supplementation of these elements is questionable, but sales of products in this class attest to their popularity.

A typical product multivitamin with minerals might contain vitamins A, C, D, E, thiamin, riboflavin, pyridoxine, sodium or calcium pantothenate, cyanocobolamine, iron, calcium, copper, magnesium, manganese, zinc, and iodine. Some members of this group have added trace elements such as selenium, chromium, molybdenum, and biotin to the formulation.

Some of the more popular multivitamins and mineral products are Centrum, One-A-Day plus Minerals, Paladac with Minerals, Stuart Formula, Unicap-M, and Vicon Plus capsules, and Viterra tablets.

Multivitamins with Iron

Dietary surveys have shown that a substantial number of Americans are deficient in iron. This has led to the development and use of a wide variety of formulas with between 10 and 18 mg. of iron per tablet or capsule. Many people believe if you need extra vitamins, you probably also need extra iron. If you accept this theory, be sure to choose a product that provides vitamins and at least 18 mg. iron. If you don't go along with this thinking, just take extra iron. The RDA of iron for all females between the ages of eleven and fifty years and for males between the ages of eleven and eighteen years. The RDA for adult men and women over the age of fifty is 10 mg.

These products are not suitable for pregnant or breastfeeding women, whose iron needs approach 60 mg. per day.

Therapeutic Multivitamins

Therapeutic formulas contain the same vitamins as those in the groups we call multivitamins and stress formulas (discussed below under "B-Complex Formulas") but in larger quantities. They can be identified by the letter *T* or the word *therapeutic* in their name. The levels of vitamins found in these formulas can approach the megadose range, ten times the RDA.

Products in this group are often recommended for older people or for those who are extremely deficient in one or two vitamins. The feeling is that, since all vitamins are obtained from food, if you are deficient in one, you are probably deficient in several others. Therefore, a therapeutic multivitamin is recommended. Most of the contents of any therapeutic formulation will either be saved in the body or eliminated via the urine, so you should consider carefully the regular use of one of these products.

Some therapeutic multivitamin products are: Theragran, Multicebrin Tablets, Stuart Therapeutic Tablets, and Fortespan Capsules. As with other multivitamins, there are low-cost versions of these formulas sold through many vitamin outlets. One of the most widely imitated formulas in this group is Theragran, and pharmacies or vitamin stores often advertise a private label brand as being "equal to Theragran."

Therapeutic Multivitamins with Minerals

Products in this class usually contain the same basic ingredients as multivitamins with minerals. The only difference is that products labeled therapeutic usually contain larger (1.5–2 times) concentrations of each ingredient. Since the extra quantities provided in the so-called therapeutic formulas are probably not necessary, the superiority of these formulations over other vitamin mixtures should be questioned.

Some of the more popular therapeutic multivitamins with minerals are: Theragran M. Mi-Cebrin T, Clusivol, and Super Plenamins Extra Strength Tablets.

Many companies have copied the Theragran M formula because of its commercial success. In fact, there are probably more Theragran M imitations than any other vitamin product. Virtually all of them are sold for less than the original product.

B-Complex Formulas

These products are usually promoted to people who want to be sure they can build red blood cells, keep their blood vessels and nervous systems functioning, and maintain normal body metabolism at a high level of efficiency.

B-complex formulas contain only the B vitamin group in quantities that approach the RDAs, although there is a tremendous range of vitamin concentrations among the various B-complex formulas. Some brands are: Geriplex-FS Liquid, Betalin Compound Pulvules (capsules), and Lederplex tablets and capsules. Some companies add a variety of other ingredients including biotin, PABA, lecithin, choline, and inositol. Despite these added ingredients, these products remain in the B-complex category.

B-Complex with C (Stress) Formulas

B-complex with C formulas were the original stress formulas. They are essentially the same B-complex vitamins but have added vitamin C.

Within the past few years, some manufacturers have updated their formulas by adding additional nutrients. The amounts of vitamins contained in most "stress formulas" exceed the RDA by several times, but the choice of ingredients and dosage strengths does not seem to follow any logical pattern.

The best-known stress formula vitamin is called Albee with C. Other brands are Stresscaps and Surbex with C.

Many manufacturers have patterned their "stress formula" after Albee with C because of its commercial success. This raises an interesting question. Obviously, people who make and sell vitamin products do so because they are interested in making money. But the promotional efforts put behind many of these products cannot be justified by their possible benefits to the consumer. Have they added extra vitamin C and other ingredients to their formulas to make their products nutritionally more complete or to keep up with the latest vitamin or mineral rage? Whenever a new ingredient is added to a vitamin product, the brand name is changed to reflect that addition. This allows the manufacturers to advertise their new, improved, complete, etc. formula. Some stress formulas to which additional nutrients, such as dessicated liver, brewer's yeast, zinc, magnesium, and folic acid, may be added are Stresstabs 600, Beminal 500, and Albee C 800.

Stress formulas are promoted for people who find themselves under tremendous stress, despite the fact that no medical evidence supports claims made for these formulas. We do use more vitamin C than normal when we are in a stressful situation, but the amount needed is far less than that found in stress formula vitamins. See the profile on vitamin C in Part II for further information on your actual needs for this vitamin.

Pediatric Vitamins

The only thing that differentiates pediatric vitamins from general multivitamins of the one-a-day variety or multivitamins with minerals is the form in which they can be purchased. The most successful pediatric products are those made and sold in the shape of animals or popular cartoon characters and flavored to taste like candy. Many children will not take vitamins unless they are flavored, can be chewed, and resemble some familiar character. So, if you want your child to take a daily multivitamin, these products may be your only choice, and there is little difference in their vitamin content.

The chewable multivitamins that have added minerals to their formulas can provide added benefits to the child who does not eat properly, but they cannot be considered a replacement for good nutrition. The latest mineral addition to children's chewable vitamins is calcium, but the amount of calcium in these products is insufficient to meet the RDA for that important mineral. Your child will still have to obtain his or her daily calcium from dietary sources. Another mineral, fluoride, is included in some formulas, and your doctor may prescribe one of these if the water supply in your area is not fluoridated.

Infants are often given a liquid product containing vitamins A, C, and D. These products are meant to supplement the vitamins supplied in infant formulas. Some pediatricians will switch the child to a more comprehensive vitamin product once the infant has stopped taking prepared formulas. Others will simply tell you to stop giving your child a vitamin on the assumption that the baby is getting all required nutrients from its food. Do not accept the doctor's recommendation on blind faith. If you know that your child is a good eater, he or she probably does not need a vitamin supplement. If, however, your child is a fussy or poor eater, he or she may need supplemental vitamins. Remember, no one knows your child better than you.

Prenatal Vitamins

The needs of the pregnant or breastfeeding woman have been studied in greater detail than those of almost any other group. Therefore, the types and amounts of micronutrients found in these formulas are more standardized than the ingredients in any other product class. Your doctor will probably recommend a specific prenatal formulation, but many different products will meet your needs. When evaluating your prenatal vitamins, bear in mind that they should meet all the RDAs specified for pregnant or lactating (breastfeeding) women. They contain more of just about every vitamin and mineral, but there are some differences among prenatal products.

All prenatal vitamins contain extra folic acid. Federal regulation allows up to 0.8 mg. a day of folic acid to be sold without a doctor's prescription. Yet a few products containing less than 0.8 mg. per pill are sold on prescription only. The vitamin manufacturer has chosen prescription-only sales because he knows that a prescription-only product can be sold for a higher price and does not have to compete on the open market; it only has to compete with other prescription products. Most prescription-only prenatal vitamins, however, contain 1 mg. of folic acid, an amount which would justify their status.

The RDAs indicate that pregnant women should be receiving at least 0.8 mg. per day of folic acid and breastfeeding women should receive 0.5 mg. Check the folic acid content of your prenatal product, since some may have as little as 0.1 mg. per pill.

Other differences among prenatal formulas to be considered are these:

• Some may be lacking in vitamin E, an essential nutrient for pregnant and breastfeeding women.
• Some prenatal vitamins don't provide enough vitamin A. Pregnant women need 1,000 mcg. (5,000 IU) every day, and those who are breastfeeding need another 200 mcg. (1,000 IU). Most are adequate, but there are a few prenatal formulas that provide only 800 mcg. (4,000 IU) per tablet.
• Mineral content varies tremendously, and some have no minerals at all.

• The amount of calcium in prenatal vitamins varies from 125 mg. to 350 mg. per pill, but none meets the RDA for calcium because of the physical difficulty of packing all that calcium into a single tablet. You must get extra calcium from milk, milk products, or some other outside source.

• Pregnant women should take between 30 and 60 mg. of iron every day. Yet some prenatal formulas provide less than 30 mg. of iron in each tablet.

• Some prenatal products have added a stool softener (to prevent you from becoming constipated) or amino acids to the basic formula (supposedly because they are part of DNA building blocks).

Geriatric Formulas

The new emphasis on geriatrics and geriatric medicine has given birth to a whole class of vitamin products marketed especially for senior citizens. But when you compare these formulas with other vitamin and mineral products, you will find that they offer no special nutritional benefit to those over age sixty-five.

There are, however, two nonnutritional features of some geriatric formulas that may be considered pluses.

Some manufacturers have incorporated a stool softener. One example is Geriplex-FS, to which docusate sodium, a fecal softener (hence the suffix ''FS'') has been added to prevent constipation while this product is being taken. Iron, an ingredient common to these and other formulas, can be constipating and particularly troublesome to anyone with bowel problems.

Another unique feature is that some geriatric vitamin formulas are sold as liquids, allowing them to be taken more easily (and at considerably greater cost per dose) by those who cannot or do not wish to swallow capsules.

If you are a senior citizen, you should consider using any vitamin-mineral formulation that meets your RDA requirements and not restrict yourself to a geriatric formula for any special nutritional benefits.

Other Formulas

Some manufacturers sell mixtures of vitamins and minerals especially for men, women, men who are losing their hair, or men with sexual potency problems. These formulas are said to be especially prepared to meet the nutritional requirements of people in each of these categories. One might ask, "Should a balding man with sexual problems take three different vitamin supplements?" Obviously, the answer to this question is a re-sounding *no!*

There is no evidence to indicate that any of these special vitamin-mineral products can produce the kind of results claimed on the package labels and in the advertising for these formulas. These formulas are excellent examples of the unsubstantiated claims which are reviewed in each vitamin and mineral profile.

Your Choice of Dosage Forms

When selecting a dosage form, you will want to pick the one that is most convenient and pleasant for you to take, while providing all of the vitamins and minerals you want. This is a very personal decision and one which can only be made by taste testing and considering the recommendations of others who have taken specific products.

All manufacturers are aware of the role that convenience, tablet size, and taste play in the selection of their products. You can be sure that each of them will strive to provide you with the best-tasting, most convenient product possible. The only axiom for you to remember here is that the larger the number of vitamins and minerals and the more of each that is contained in a tablet, the larger the tablet. That's why so many of the new, all-inclusive products, the ones with everything under the sun, are large enough to be considered true "horse pills." Here is a brief rundown of the most common dosage forms.

Tablets and Capsules

Most vitamins are sold as tablets or capsules simply because this is the most convenient way for manufacturers to pack all those nutrients into a single dosage unit. Other dosage forms usually contain less nutrient per dosage unit.

Chewable Tablets

These are special formulas for young children and others

who cannot swallow traditional tablets or capsules. They are comparable to multivitamin, multivitamin with minerals, or multivitamin with iron products. The major differences among these products lie in their taste and shape, both of which may be important to the person actually chewing and swallowing the product.

Liquids

Liquid vitamin products were originally developed as another convenience for people who are unable to swallow tablets or capsules. Generally they contain relatively small amounts of nutrients in a dosage unit—usually a teaspoon or tablespoon. This is because vitamins can be difficult to dissolve and are unpalatable to some people even at modest dosage ranges. Most liquid vitamins contain a healthy dose of alcohol, needed to dissolve some of the vitamins.

Powders

If you're a purist, then vitamin powders would be for you. However, your total daily vitamin and mineral needs would just about fill a teaspoon, so it would be relatively impractical for you to measure daily doses of supplemental vitamins and minerals. In fact, the only vitamin sold widely in powder form is C, and this grew out of the practice of taking megadoses in the range of 5–10 g. per day for the common cold.

Wafers and Other Food Products

A few vitamins are available as wafers or other food products. These are simply more convenient ways for people to take a vitamin supplement. There is even a breakfast cereal, Total, which has enough vitamin content to meet 100 percent of the adult U.S. RDA of each ingredient. The manufacturers of that product have used that fact as a major part of their advertising campaign.

Taking Vitamins and Minerals: When and How

Vitamins and minerals may be taken at any time, without

regard to meal time. The body will extract everything it needs, regardless of dosage form or time of day.

Sometimes, however, food can be helpful in affecting the rate of absorption of minerals, such as iron. In these cases, the food delays the passage of the mineral through the intestines and allows more time for the mineral to be absorbed into your bloodstream through the intestinal tissues. Also, food may reduce the chances of getting an upset stomach from vitamins or vitamin-mineral combinations that you may find irritating or upsetting.

It is a good idea to get into the habit of taking your vitamins at the same time every day; this establishes a routine and helps you to remember to take them. Many people take their vitamins with breakfast; others prefer lunch time, coffee break, or bedtime.

Vitamin and Mineral Interactions

Most vitamins and minerals at doses near the RDA values do not significantly affect the absorption of other vitamins and minerals. Sometimes, though, one nutrient will help another to be absorbed into the blood. For example, vitamin C assists in the absorption of iron. In contrast, vitamin E, in large doses, has been reported to counteract the effects of iron in treating infant anemia. Don't give your child large doses of E unless instructed to do so by your pediatrician.

Additional vitamin-mineral interactions as well as interactions of both with medications are detailed in Part IV, "Vitamin, Mineral and Drug Interactions."

Vitamins and Government Control

Government regulation of the manufacture and sale of vitamins and minerals lies with the U.S. Food and Drug Administration (FDA). At the present time they are regulated as food products, although the agency has attempted several times over the years to change the classification of these nutrient products to "special foods," at first, and then to drugs.

As it now stands, the FDA's role in regard to vitamins and minerals is limited to two areas: the agency can set controls to protect public safety, and it can challenge claims that are demonstrably outrageous. This is in contrast to drugs, where the FDA has control not only over safety but also over *effectiveness*.

Two important rulings concerning vitamins and safety were made during the 1970s. In 1973, the FDA was able to limit the sale of vitamins A and D to dosages the agency judged safe for unsupervised use by the general public. You cannot buy products containing individual doses of vitamin A larger than 2 mg. (2,000 mcg. or 10,000 IU) or of vitamin D larger than 10 mcg. (400 IU) without a prescription from your doctor. And a 1976 amendment to the Federal Food, Drug, and Cosmetic Act gave the agency control over vitamins and minerals made for pregnant and breastfeeding women, for children under age twelve and for adults in instances where the agency was able to demonstrate toxic effects from the product. These regulations were revoked in 1978 after prolonged litigation. Unfortunately there are now no restrictions on vitamin potencies. Let the buyer beware!

There is, in effect, relatively little control over the methods vitamin and mineral manufacturers can use to try and convince you to buy and use their products. This is, in our opinion, an unfortunate situation because it fosters outright quackery and may prevent a consumer from getting the true story about vitamins and minerals he or she may be buying as part of an overall health maintenance program.

Table 8

Contents of Top-Selling Multivitamin Products

Product (Manufacturer)	Vitamin A(IU)	Vitamin D(IU)	Vitamin E(IU)	C(mg.)	B₁(mg.)	B₂(mg.)	B₆(mg.)	Niacin (mg.)	B₁₂(mg.)	Pantothenic Acid (mg.)	Iron (mg.)	Calcium (mg.)	Other
Multiple vitamins													
Albee with C (Robins)	0	0	0	300	15.00	10.0	5.0	50	0	10.0	0	0	
Albee C-800 (Robins)	0	0	45	800	15.00	17.0	25.0	100	12	25.0	0	0	
Beminal 500 (Ayerst)	0	0	0	500	25.00	12.5	10.0	100	5	0	0	20	
Cebefortis (Upjohn)	0	0	0	150	5.00	5.0	1.0	50	2	10.0	0	0	
One-A-Day (Miles)	5,000	400	15	60	1.50	1.7	2.0	20	6	0	0	0	Folic acid 400 mcg.
Surbex (Abbott)	0	0	0	0	6.00	6.0	2.5	30	5	10.0	0	0	
Theragran (Squibb)	10,000	400	15	200	10.30	10.0	4.1	100	5	21.4	0	0	
Unicap (Upjohn)	5,000	400	15	60	1.50	1.7	2.0	20	6	0	0	0	Folic acid 400 mcg.
Stresscaps (Lederle)	0	0	0	300	10.00	10.0	2.0	100	4	20.0	0	0	

84

Multiple vitamins plus iron and minerals

Product													Additional minerals
Centrum (Lederle)	5,000	400	30	90	2.25	2.6	3.0	20	9	10.0	27	162	Folic acid 400 mcg. Phosphorous 125 mg. Magnesium 100 mg. Potassium 7.5 mg. Iodine 150 mcg. Zinc 22.5 mg.
Myadec (Parke-Davis)	10,000	400	30	250	10.00	10.0	5.0	100	6	20.0	20	0	Folic acid 400 mcg. Magnesium 100 mg. Zinc 20 mg. Iodine 150 mcg.
Theragran-M (Squibb)	10,000	400	15	200	10.00	10.0	4.1	100	5	20.0	12	0	Magnesium 65 mg. Zinc 1.5 mg. Iodine 150 mcg.

Product (Manufacturer)	Vitamin A(IU)	Vitamin D(IU)	Vitamin E(IU)	C(mg.)	B₁(mg.)	B₂(mg.)	B₆(mg.)	Niacin (mg.)	B₁₂(mg.)	Pantothenic Acid (mcg.)	Iron (mg.)	Calcium (mg.)	Other
Therapeutic vitamins plus iron and minerals													
Unicap T (Upjohn)	5,000	400	15	300	10.00	10.0	6.0	100	18	10.0	18	0	Folic acid 400 mcg. Potassium 5.0 mg. Iodine 150 mcg. Zinc 15 mg.
Gevral T (Lederle)	5,000	400	45	90	2.25	2.6	3.0	30	9	0	27	162	Folic acid 400 mcg. Potassium 5.0 mg. Zinc 22.5 mg. Iodine 22.5 mcg.
Multiple vitamins with iron													
Albee C-800 plus Iron (Robins)	0	0	45	800	15.00	17.0	25.0	100	12	25.0	0	0	Folic acid 400 mcg.

Product												Other
Cebetinic (Upjohn)	0	0	25	2.00	2.0	0.5	10	5	0	38	0	
Geritol (Miles)	0	0	75	5.00	5.0	0.5	30	3	2.0	50	0	
Surbex 750 with Iron (Abbott)	0	30	750	15.00	15.0	25.0	100	12	20.0	27	0	Folic acid 400 mcg.
Pediatric vitamins												
Bugs Bunny (Miles)	2,500	15	60	1.05	1.2	1.05	13.5	4.5	0	0	0	Folic acid 300 mcg.
Flintstones (Miles)	2,500	15	60	1.05	1.2	1.05	13.5	4.5	0	0	0	Folic acid 300 mcg.
Pediatric vitamins plus iron												
Geritol Jr. Tablets (J.B. Williams)	5,000	15	30	2.50	2.5	1.00	20.0	1.0	2	25	0	
Poly-Vi-Sol with Iron Chew (Mead Johnson)	2,500	15	60	1.05	1.2	7.50	13.5	50.0	15	100	0	Folic acid 50 mcg. Docusate 100 mg. (stool softener)
Pediatric vitamin drops												
Poly-Vi-Sol (Mead Johnson)	1,500	5	35	0.50	0.6	0.40	8.0	0	0	0	0	

Product (Manufacturer)	Vitamin A(IU)	Vitamin D(IU)	Vitamin E(IU)	C(mg.)	B1(mg.)	B2(mg.)	B6(mg.)	Niacin (mg.)	B12(mg.)	Pantothenic Acid (mcg.)	Iron (mg.)	Calcium (mg.)	Other
Pediatric drops plus iron Poly-Vi-Sol with Iron (Mead Johnson)	1,500	400	5	35	0.50	0.6	0.40	8.0	0	0	10	0	0
Prenatal multiple vitamins Stuart Prenatal (Stuart)	8,000	400	30	60	1.70	2.0	4.00	20.0	8.0	0	60	200	Folic acid 800 mcg. Magnesium 100 mg. Iodine 15 mcg.
Natalins (Mead Johnson)	8,000	400	30	90	1.70	2.0	4.00	20.0	8.0	0	45	200	Folic acid 800 mcg. Magnesium 100 mg. Iodine 150 mcg.

Part II

VITAMIN PROFILES

7

Water-Soluble Vitamins

Vitamin B$_1$
Thiamin

Popularly known as the "energy vitamin," thiamin is actually one of several B-complex vitamins involved in metabolic processes essential to the release of energy.

The discovery of thiamin is closely tied to a debilitating disease—beriberi—which has been known since antiquity but suddenly reached epidemic proportions in the Orient in the nineteenth century. Not coincidentally, it was at that time that the practice of polishing rice was introduced. As the vitamin-rich covering of rice was removed, people who relied on this food as a staple were unwittingly deprived of essential thiamin.

It was not until the 1930s that the substance that can prevent beriberi—now known as thiamin—was discovered in the residue of rice polishings. Once the chemical structure of thiamin was determined, a process for making it synthetically was developed, and today virtually all the thiamin we take is manufactured.

Function

Thiamin is primarily involved in the metabolism of carbo-hydrates (sugars) in the body. The process of carbohydrate metabolism is quite complex, and thiamin is a factor in three separate parts of that process. In each case, thiamin acts as a coenzyme (or catalyst). Coenzymes are agents that speed or enable a chemical reaction to occur but are not participants in that chemical reaction.

The first reaction for which thiamin acts as a coenzyme is called glycolysis. In glycolysis, sugars are converted to energy. In effect, glycolysis can be compared to putting logs on a fire. Without thiamin, we would not be able to release the energy from glucose; we would not be able to burn the logs. The actual enzyme helped by thiamin is called pyruvate dehydrogenase. Pyruvate dehydrogenase links the chemical reactions that split large sugars into small ones and the reactions that burn the smaller sugars.

Second, thiamin is involved in the reactions that burn the smaller sugars produced by glycolysis. This, in turn, involves several different chemical reactions and is commonly known as the Krebs cycle. In the Krebs cycle, thiamin acts as a coenzyme for an enzyme called alpha ketoglutarate dehydrogenase. If thiamin were not present, this enzyme could not function and you would not be able to live because you could not use carbohydrate (sugar) energy efficiently.

The third reaction in which thiamin is a coenzyme involves an enzyme called transketolase. Transketolase cannot function unless thiamin is present. It is involved in the production of ribose and NADP, two chemicals essential to the operation of every cell in the body because they are ingredients in the manufacture of the nucleic acids. Nucleic acids are the basis of your genes, which control all cell and body functions.

In addition, thiamin is involved in the transmission of nerve impulses throughout the body. We can conclude that thiamin is involved in chemical reactions that provide energy to nerve cells, but its exact role in this process is not known.

Daily Requirements

Daily thiamin requirements depend on the number of calories taken in on an average day. You need 0.5 mg. for every 1,000 calories of energy. If you normally eat about 3,000 calories, your daily requirement is about 1.5 mg.; if you only eat 2,000 calories, your requirement is reduced to 1 mg.

People who normally expend large amounts of energy, such as athletes and construction workers, and those who normally take in a high carbohydrate diet should consider the need to supplement their thiamin intake, according to the amount of energy involved.

Dietary Sources

Fortunately, small amounts of thiamin are present in nearly all living things. Most Americans get their dietary thiamin from enriched flour, whole grains, and lean beef. Additional good sources are listed in the accompanying table.

Thiamin is stable when frozen and stored. When heated, thiamin is also stable in fruits and foods that are processed in acidic solutions such as vinegar. However, prolonged cooking of meats and vegetables, which are "basic," or nonacidic, can destroy significant amounts of thiamin. For example, roasting meat destroys 30–50 percent of its thiamin content, and canning or boiling vegetables destroys up to 40 percent of the thiamin present. Certainly, we are not suggesting that everyone eat raw vegetables and meat, but rather that you pay attention to your total daily thiamin intake, assuming an approximate loss of 50 percent for cooking and processing. If you cannot obtain fresh-cooked—preferably steamed—vegetables, you can minimize your thiamin losses by eating vegetables pickled in vinegar or frozen.

If you eat large amounts of raw clams and fish, you should be aware of an enzyme called thiaminase, which destroys thiamin in raw seafood but is itself destroyed in cooking. This interaction is becoming more important because of the increased popularity in America of seafood in the form of sushi and sashimi.

VITAMIN B₁ (THIAMIN) CONTENT OF SELECTED FOODS

Average adult RDA is 1.2 mg.

Food	Approximate Content (mg. per 3 oz.)
Beans	0.60
Beef	0.60
Brazil nuts	0.85
Brewer's yeast	1.60
Chickpeas	0.30
Corn	0.33
Eggs	0.16
Figs (dried)	0.90
Gooseberries (raw)	0.15
Liver	0.22
Oats	0.60
Pork	0.60
Peas	0.72
Peanuts	1.20
Pecans	0.79
Potatoes	0.10
Rice (enriched)	0.30
Rice (whole)	0.45
Rice bran	2.30
Sesame seeds	0.90
Soybeans	1.10
Sunflower seeds	2.20
Wheat germ*	20.00
White flour (enriched)	0.50
Whole wheat flour	0.50

*3 oz. of wheat germ is equivalent to about 18 teaspoons.

Deficiencies

Given the role that thiamin plays in sugar metabolism, it will come as no surprise that thiamin deficiency can be dangerous and life threatening.

In the United States and England, refined white flour is, by law, enriched with thiamin (as well as riboflavin and nicotinic acid). Thus, even though most of the original B vitamin content of the flour is removed during processing, white flour represents an important source of dietary thiamin, and gross thiamin deficiencies are relatively uncommon where enriched white flour is used. Marginal thiamin deficiencies are much more common and usually associated with inattention to proper diet.

Symptoms of Deficiency

Early signs of marginal thiamin deficiency include loss of appetite—which only aggravates the problem of thiamin deficiency—and weight loss, vomiting, nausea, weakness, fatigue, and mental problems such as rolling of the eyeballs, depression, memory loss, difficulty concentrating and dealing with details, and personality changes.

Gross thiamin deficiency results in the classical disease, beriberi, which takes three forms: cardiac (affecting the heart); central nervous system (affecting brain and nerve function); and gastrointestinal (affecting the stomach and intestines). The symptoms of each vary tremendously with the degree of deficiency, age of the patient, and speed with which the disease developed. Disease with more rapid onset is usually more serious. Physical signs of gross thiamin deficiency include muscle weakness, decreased reflex activity, fluid in the arms and legs, enlargement of the heart, nausea and vomiting, and nervous system problems similar to those associated with marginal deficiency.

Thiamin function can be tested in two ways. One is a relatively simple blood test your doctor can order called transketolase function after the fact that the activity of the transketolase enzyme is directly related to levels of thiamin in the body. The other involves the level of pyruvic acid in the blood; people with a thiamin deficiency will have more pyruvic acid in their blood because of the changes in sugar metabolism that occur when sufficient thiamin is not present.

Thiamin and Alcoholics

The alcoholic patient presents a special problem when it comes to thiamin. Not only is his or her diet deficient in thiamin, but alcohol interferes with the passage of what little thiamin is eaten in foodstuffs into the bloodstream. Alcohol may even cause thiamin to be displaced from sites in the body where it is needed. Ironically, alcoholics need more thiamin than the average person because of their very high carbohydrate intake (alcohol is a carbohydrate). They need the thiamin to push forward the metabolism and utilization of all that extra carbohydrate.

A nerve disease called Wernicke-Korsakoff syndrome may occur in alcoholics as a result of their severe drinking and thiamin deficiency. There is also evidence that alcoholics have a genetic tendency toward this condition. People with Wernicke-Korsakoff show symptoms of confusion, memory loss, and psychotic behavior, and some symptoms may remain even after the vitamin deficiency has been corrected. The cost of institutionalizing and treating Wernicke-Korsakoff patients has been estimated at more than $70 million per year in the United States alone, and it has therefore been suggested that small amounts of thiamin be added to alcoholic beverages to prevent the development of this syndrome. We believe this approach should be given serious consideration.

Thiamin and Diabetics

Diabetics who have marginal thiamin deficiencies may develop a mild form of Wernicke-Korsakoff syndrome when taking their antidiabetes medicines. The treatment of diabetes is aimed at reducing high blood sugar levels by providing extra insulin or stimulating the pancreas to make more insulin. Once the insulin gets into the blood, it stimulates the metabolism of glucose by the normal pathways which involve thiamin. If the diabetic is already marginally thiamin deficient, this process can accentuate the deficiency symptoms and, in a few cases, has resulted in the development of Wernicke-Korsakoff syndrome. Diabetics can avoid this situation simply by taking a daily multivitamin or eating foods known to be rich in thiamin content.

Thiamin and Other Special Groups

Others who should pay special attention to their thiamin intake in order to avoid deficiencies are senior citizens, who have been shown to be consistently deficient in thiamin, and pregnant and lactating women, whose thiamin requirements are significantly greater because of their increased energy expenditure.

Toxicity

Few reports of adverse reactions to thiamin have been noted in the medical literature. Thiamin is generally considered to be safe and nontoxic when taken by mouth; injections have resulted in a few allergic reactions, but life-threatening situations are rarely encountered.

A small number of animal studies, however, have revealed that administration of large amounts of thiamin over a prolonged period of time interferes with the animals' ability to eliminate some drugs and, perhaps, cancer-causing chemicals. The importance of this observation to people who regularly consume excess amounts of thiamin is not known, but our advice, as presented throughout this book, is that long-term consumption of large amounts of *any* vitamin is ill advised unless there are specific therapeutic reasons for doing so.

Interactions

Thiamin can interact with drugs used to relax muscles during surgery to produce excessive muscle relaxation, but no special precautions are needed.

Therapeutic Uses

Thiamin supplements may be given to counteract any of the symptoms of thiamin deficiency reviewed earlier in this profile. However, such symptoms will not be alleviated by thiamin unless they are, in fact, caused by vitamin deficiency.

In addition, thiamin can be used to treat certain rare metabolic defects present in small numbers of people in which the thiamin dependent enzymes discussed under "Function" are abnormal and require inordinately large amounts of the vitamin.

These so-called inborn errors are often first discovered in infants or children who exhibit learning disabilities. These disabilities develop because insufficient amounts of energy are provided to a developing nervous system. If the infant or child is

97

treated with thiamin early and vigorously, the condition may improve dramatically. However, thiamin is not helpful in treating any other kinds of learning disabilities.

Unsubstantiated Claims

Nerve Tonic

Thiamin had been used as a cure-all nerve tonic for many years when modern researchers finally determined its ineffectiveness for this purpose. Yet the popularity of thiamin as a nerve tonic continues, solely because of individual testimonials and word-of-mouth endorsements. Also, vitamin manufacturers and marketers are still free to promote their products for this and other questionable uses because vitamins are not as tightly regulated as drugs.

The usual thought process goes like this: if nervous system problems are a consequence of thiamin deficiency, thiamin must be a good treatment for all nerve problems, regardless of their origin. Obviously, this is fuzzy thinking. Thiamin can help only if the nerve problems are actually caused by thiamin deficiency.

Insect Repellant

Another invalid application of thiamin that has achieved increasing popularity among consumers over the past several years is its use as an insect repellant. The popularity of thiamin for this purpose stems from several isolated reports of successful use in medical literature. The theory is that if you take large amounts of thiamin by mouth, insects will be repelled by the unpleasant taste and odor of thiamin in the perspiration. Therefore, they may swarm but will not bite. Despite the fact that careful studies of this claim have failed to prove its value—and the fact that the Food and Drug Administration determined that thiamin is ineffective as a repellant in January 1982—some dermatologists continue to recommand one 150 mg. tablet of thiamin three or four times every day you will be exposed, beginning one day before you go into the woods. A dose in this range would probably not cause any harm, despite the fact that it approaches 100 times the average adult RDA of thiamin. It is just unlikely to work as an insect repellant.

Thiamin has also been promoted for other uses for which its value has not been proven. We cannot recommend that you take this vitamin to treat motion sickness or pain. Thiamin will also not improve appetite, digestion, or mental alertness, nor will it promote growth.

Availability

Thiamin tablets are available without a prescription in strengths of 5 mg., 10 mg., 25 mg., 250 mg., and 500 mg. Thiamin elixir (Bewon Elixir) can also be bought without a prescription and contains 0.25 mg. in every teaspoonful. Thiamin injection requires a prescription from your doctor.

Vitamin B₂
Riboflavin

The presence of riboflavin is easily detected by its yellow color and somewhat unpleasant taste. In fact, the distinct taste of multivitamin preparations is due to riboflavin content.

Like most B-complex vitamins, riboflavin is involved with energy production. But unlike the others, a lack of this vitamin manifests itself primarily in skin sores and blemishes that affect not only the outer skin but the lining of the stomach.

Function

Riboflavin is converted in the body to two active forms, flavin mononucleotide (FMN) and flavin adenine dinucleotide (FAD). FMN and FAD are essential to cell function because they are coenzymes (catalysts) for chemical reactions that involve utilization of oxygen and liberation of energy. The energy that is released is used by each cell to convert food into more energy, which it then uses to perform its designated functions in the body. Riboflavin is found in every cell in the body.

Daily Requirements

As is the case with thiamin, the daily requirement of riboflavin can be related to the number of calories you take in each day. The more calories, the more riboflavin you will need to convert food to useful energy. It is generally accepted that you should be getting 0.6 mg. of riboflavin for every 1,000 calories you eat. Therefore, if you are on a 3,000-calorie diet, you will need 1.8 mg., if you eat 2,000 calories, you will need only 1.2 mg., and so on.

People who expend large amounts of energy every day should take care to supplement their daily riboflavin intake. Athletes, construction workers, and others with heavy daily physical demands fall into this category.

Dietary Sources

Proteins combined with riboflavin—called flavoproteins—are important to all forms of life. It is therefore logical that riboflavin is found in a wide variety of foods. Particularly rich sources are milk, cheese, chicken, lean beef, and pork. Additional good sources are listed in the accompanying table.

Riboflavin is stable when heated, and because it is not as soluble in water as some of the other vitamins, much of the vitamin content of foods cooked in water (about 80 percent) is retained in the finished product, even if the cooking water is discarded. Riboflavin is destroyed when mixed with basic substances, such as baking soda.

However, riboflavin is broken down by sunlight; you should therefore keep riboflavin-rich substances away from direct sunlight. Normal room lights are not strong enough to cause much riboflavin destruction, although common sense would dictate that dark or opaque containers be used for cooking and storage in order to minimize vitamin losses. Placing clear milk bottles on a sunny porch may be picturesque, but it destroys most of the riboflavin content. This is particularly unfortunate because milk is one of the most important dietary sources of this vitamin.

Grains contain most of their riboflavin in the germ and bran coat; therefore, bleaching and other refining processes used to produce white flour remove most of this vitamin from this important dietary staple. In "enriched" flour, riboflavin as well

Vitamin B₂ (Riboflavin) Content of Selected Foods
Average adult RDA is 1.2 mg.

Food	Approximate content (mg. per 3 oz.)
Almonds	0.81
Apricots (dried)	0.15
Bee pollen	1.70
Beans	0.20
Boysenberries (frozen)	0.11
Brewer's yeast	3.40*
Broccoli	0.18
Cheese	0.43
Chicken	0.34
Corn	0.17
Cottage cheese	0.23
Cream cheese	0.13
Dates (pitted)	0.09
Eggs	0.17
Liver	3.60
Meats (lean beef and pork)	0.17
Milk	0.15
Mushrooms	0.30
Mustard greens	0.60
Parsley	0.23
Passion fruit	0.12
Pears (dried)	0.16
Peas	0.23
Prunes (dried)	0.20
Raspberries (red or black)	0.08
Spinach	0.17
Sprouts	0.17
Strawberries	0.07
Turkey	0.18
Veal	0.28
Wheat germ	0.60
White flour	0.05
White flour (enriched)	0.13
Whole wheat flour	0.13
Yogurt	0.16

*Equivalent to 18 teaspoons.

as thiamin and niacin have been added to replace the amounts removed in processing. Enriched is better than nonenriched, but it makes more sense to eat the unadulterated, vitamin-complete, whole grain when possible.

Deficiencies

Riboflavin deficiency may be difficult to recognize because it rarely occurs alone. It is normally accompanied by other vitamin deficiencies and is most commonly encountered among people whose diets are inadequate or consist mostly of carbohydrates.

A person who consumes insufficient amounts of protein will force the body to break down its own proteins, including the riboflavin-containing flavoproteins. Thus, a severely low protein diet will lead to a riboflavin deficiency unless unusually large amounts of the vitamin are obtained from dietary or other sources, an unlikely prospect if protein intake is so low.

Considering the importance of riboflavin-dependent enzymes to energy production and body metabolic processes, it is remarkable that riboflavin deficiencies are not more serious and life threatening. The reasons for this are not well understood but may be due to the widespread availability of riboflavin from foods; it would be very difficult to consume a riboflavin-free diet.

Symptoms of Deficiency

There are groups of symptoms known to accompany riboflavin deficiency, and many of these symptoms can be traced to a general loss of ability to perform normal tissue repairs.

The first symptoms are a general loss of facial color, sores at the corner of the mouth, and a sore throat. These may be followed by a magenta coloration of the tongue called glossitis, red and raw lips, and skin sores (especially in cracks and around joints). A greasy, scaling rash may develop between the nose and face and can spread to involve both cheeks and the skin around the ears. Rashes in the genital area are common. People with severe riboflavin deficiency may become anemic or develop nerve disease, but these are relatively infrequent.

One interesting feature of riboflavin deficiency is the invasion of blood vessels into the cornea of the eye with a resultant appearance that can be compared to "red eye," or conjunctivitis. The eye, in contrast to other organs, does not contain FMN or FAD. Rather, it contains free riboflavin. It is thought that free riboflavin in the eye may play a role in bringing oxygen to those tissues which have no other obvious sources of oxygen. When there is not enough riboflavin in the eye, the body compensates by causing blood vessels to grow into the normally clear cornea to supply needed oxygen.

Riboflavin level is best tested by measuring the amount of vitamin passed out of the urine over a twenty-four-hour period. People who lose less than 0.05 mg. per twenty-four-hour period are probably deficient. People with riboflavin anemias will also begin to make new red blood cells and will experience an increase in blood hemoglobin level after taking the vitamin. This effect can be monitored by routine blood counts and hemoglobin levels. In addition, people who are riboflavin deficient may have low levels of an enzyme in red blood cells called glutathione reductase.

Riboflavin and Special Groups

Severe riboflavin deficiencies are rare in the United States, but marginal deficiencies involving many of the symptoms described above have been observed in alcoholics. Also, dietary surveys have revealed marginal deficiencies in some senior citizens, the poor, and some urban teenagers who do not drink milk regularly.

Pregnant and breastfeeding women need extra riboflavin because of their increased energy requirements.

Drugs and Riboflavin Deficiency

Scientists have noted that women taking oral contraceptives (The Pill) or thyroid hormones may be riboflavin deficient. Also, animal studies indicate that those who take phenothiazine (antipsychotic) drugs such as chlorpromazine (Thorazine and others), tricyclic antidepressants such as amitryptilline (Elavil and others), may have less riboflavin in their bodies than people not taking those medicines. The reasons for this are not known.

Toxicity

Riboflavin is not considered to be toxic, and excess riboflavin is rapidly passed out of the body via the urine. Those who favor consumption of large doses of the B vitamins need only look at the bright yellow color of their urine—due to riboflavin—to appreciate how much of their "megadose" is being flushed down the toilet.

Therapeutic Uses

Riboflavin supplements may be given to counteract any of the symptoms of riboflavin deficiency reviewed earlier in this profile. However, such symptoms will not be alleviated by riboflavin unless they are, in fact, caused by vitamin deficiency.

Riboflavin has no significant therapeutic use other than relief or prevention of the deficiency state.

Unsubstantiated Claims

Cure for Skin and Eye Diseases

The use of riboflavin to cure "red eye" caused by vitamin deficiency has led to the use of riboflavin in doses of 5–10 mg. per day to prevent or even cure various eye diseases. Riboflavin has also been used to treat skin disorders that mimic those seen in people with riboflavin deficiencies. These uses for riboflavin were popular in the 1940s but have fallen into disfavor more recently. Unfortunately, riboflavin only works in skin and eye diseases when the reason for the disorder is the lack of riboflavin.

Riboflavin has also been promoted for other uses for which its value has not been proven. B_2 will not prevent cancer or stress, improve reproduction, or increase growth.

Availability

Riboflavin is available from various manufacturers as tablets in strengths of 5 mg., 10 mg., 25 mg., 50 mg., and 100 mg. Riboflavin is also available on prescription only as a solution for injection containing 50 mg. per ml. It is also an ingredient in most multivitamin products.

Vitamin B$_3$
Nicotinic Acid/Niacin

Nicotinic acid is frequently called niacin, and the two terms are synonymous; however, technically speaking, nicotinic acid is the basic unit and niacin a derivative. Nicotinamide (also called niacinamide) is a close chemical cousin of nicotinic acid and is, in fact, another form of vitamin B$_3$. For practical purposes, all three forms of B$_3$ have equal vitamin activity.

On the surface, nicotinic acid appears similar to thiamin, vitamin B$_1$, but the two vitamins are actually involved in energy metabolism in somewhat different ways.

The discovery of nicotinic acid was triggered by epidemics of pellagra in the South in the early 1900s. The heavily corn-based diet then prevalent in that area was lacking in nicotinic acid and led to this debilitating and sometimes fatal deficiency disease. It has virtually disappeared in the United States since white flour began to be enriched with nicotinic acid in 1939.

Contrary to what you might think, nicotinic acid is not related to nicotine, as the name might imply.

Function

Nicotinic acid must be converted to nicotinamide adenine dinucleotide (NAD) or nicotinamide adenine dinucleotide phosphate (NADP) before it can exert a physiologic effect. Both NAD and NADP serve as coenzymes (catalysts) for more than 150 different cellular reactions involved in generating energy for normal cell function. Nicotinic acid may also be involved in the processes by which skin pigments are made.

Daily Requirements

The daily requirement of nicotinic acid is related to the number of calories taken in and the amount of energy expended each day. At least 4.4 mg. of nicotinic acid is required for every 1,000 calories of energy expended to prevent pellagra, but the RDA is set at 6.6 mg. for every 1,000 calories. Under no circumstances should your daily intake fall below 13 mg., regardless of the number of calories you take in.

People who expend large amounts of energy on a regular basis should consider taking extra nicotinic acid to provide for that energy. Construction workers, athletes, laborers, and others with physical occupations fall into this category.

Dietary Sources

The body obtains nicotinic acid from dietary sources in two ways: it gets pure nicotinic acid from foods containing that substance; and it makes nicotinic acid from a chemical known as tryptophan, also found in many foods. However, you must take in 60 mg. of tryptophan in order to make the equivalent of 1 mg. of nicotinic acid. In addition, the chemical reactions involved in converting tryptophan to nicotinic acid require the chemical pyridoxine (vitamin B_6) to be present as a coenzyme (catalyst).

Most people receive about half their daily nicotinic acid requirement as the pure vitamin and make the rest from tryptophan. Fortunately, nicotinic acid and/or tryptophan are present in a wide variety of foods, and this makes it relatively easy to satisfy nicotinic acid requirement by dietary means. Some rich sources of this vitamin are liver, turkey, tuna, and peanuts. Nicotinic acid is also present in coffee and beer, but you would have to drink a quart of coffee or twenty-five to thirty bottles of beer a day to reach the RDA!

Additional good sources are listed in the accompanying table. There the nicotinic acid content of foods is expressed in terms of nicotinic acid *equivalents*. Thus, you don't have to think about the food content of tryptophan versus nicotinic acid; that has already been taken into consideration.

Nicotinic acid is very stable when heated or stored over long periods of time. However, this vitamin is highly water soluble and will pass into cooking water, where it will be lost if the cooking water is discarded.

Deficiencies

Nicotinic acid deficiency has been particularly noted in areas of the world where daily protein intake consists primarily of corn or other cereals that are poor sources of both tryptophan and nicotinic acid.

Vitamin B₃ Nicotinic Acid/Niacin
Content of Selected Foods

Average adult RDA is 16 mg. All concentrations of nicotinic acid are expressed as the *equivalent* content of nicotinic acid.

Food	Approximate Content (mg. per 3 oz.)
Almonds	3.15
Barley	3.33
Beef	4.24
Brewer's yeast	32.30*
Halibut	8.28
Liver	13.60
Mushrooms	3.80
Peaches (dried)	4.76
Peanuts	14.45
Pork	5.00
Potatoes	4.40
Rice, brown	4.30
Rice, white	3.25
Salmon	11.70
Sardines	4.90
Shrimp	3.00
Sprouts	2.55
Swordfish	10.00
Sunflower seeds	5.00
Tunafish	10.20
Turkey	9.35
Wheat	3.87
White flour	3.65
Whole wheat flour	3.65
Veal	7.00

*Equivalent to approximately 18 teaspoons.

Other conditions that can contribute to the development of nicotinic acid deficiency are gastrointestinal problems that interfere with the body's ability to absorb the vitamin, unusual dietary habits, infections, an overactive thyroid, and other stressful situations. Since nicotinic acid is related to the production of energy, it is also easy to understand how any condition that places extra stress on the body or demands the expenditure of energy will increase the need for nicotinic acid.

Nicotinic acid deficiency may develop in people with a rare disease called carcinoid syndrome, even though there is no problem with vitamin intake. In carcinoid syndrome, tumors develop that make large amounts of chemicals called 5-hydroxy-tryptophan and 5-hydroxytryptamine. The tumors use dietary tryptophan to make these chemicals and force the development of a vitamin deficiency. Deficiency can also develop in people with another rare condition called Hartnup's disease, which is a natural inability to absorb tryptophan from the gut.

Symptoms of Deficiency

Symptoms of the classic nicotinic acid deficiency state called pellagra can be summarized by reviewing the "four Ds": dermatitis, diarrhea, dementia, and death.

Dermatitis (skin rash) is the most distinguishing feature of pellagra. The rash appears as scaling, flaking skin, and in more severe cases, cracking and bleeding occur. It is usually located in areas where skin is stressed, such as the elbows, feet, hands, and areas of skin exposed to the sun, and the exposed areas become noticeably darker than other areas of skin. Casal's Necklace, one of the best-known signs of niacin deficiency, consists of darkening of the skin on face, neck, and back, and it appears as if the victim were wearing a dark necklace.

The diarrhea of pellagra can be quite severe and will further aggravate the problem. It can cause loss of appetite, reducing still further the absorption of nicotinic acid from foodstuffs. The diarrhea is probably caused by lesions in the stomach and intestinal tract caused by the vitamin deficiency. Other symptoms involving the gastrointestinal tract are upset and irritated stomach, a red and swollen tongue with sores on it, and enlarged salivary glands that produce excess saliva. Nausea and vomiting are common, and about half of the people who develop pellagra also lose their digestive juices until the disorder is corrected.

Dementia, the third "D," is an unusual feature of vitamin deficiency and may be simply defined as a serious mental impairment with disorientation. If untreated, the dementia can progress to the point where the victim enters a catatonic state and will die in a coma. Other symptoms of nicotinic acid deficiency involving the brain and central nervous system are irritability, memory loss, anxiety, hallucinations, and delirium.

Not all people who are deficient in nicotinic acid will develop pellagra. The most common symptoms of marginal deficiency, also known as subclinical pellagra, are diarrhea, headaches, nervousness, and a swollen and red tongue.

The only way to test for a nicotinic acid deficiency is to measure the level in your urine of methylnicotinamide—final product of the body's metabolism of nicotinic acid. Low levels of this substance indicate a possible vitamin deficiency, but the test result is not always conclusive.

Niacin and Special Groups

Alcoholics, pregnant and breastfeeding women, people with infections or overactive thyroid, and those under a great deal of daily stress may become deficient and should consider a routine nicotinic acid supplement.

Women taking oral contraceptives (the Pill) require more than 60 mg. of tryptophan to make the equivalent of 1 mg. of nicotinic acid because their conversion rate is reduced. They should increase intake of foods high in nicotinic acid or take a nutritional supplement.

Toxicity

Problems should not be encountered if doses up to 100 mg. per day are taken. However, patients taking more than 500 mg. per day of nicotinic acid will experience significant adverse reactions to that therapy.

Virtually everyone taking these high doses becomes flushed within two hours of taking the vitamin. The flush is usually confined to face and hands and can be described as burning, redness, and stinging. Tolerance to this reaction develops in time so that it becomes less severe as time goes on.

In addition, many people experience stomach upset, cramps, nausea, vomiting, and diarrhea. Liver damage can also be caused by nicotinic acid, if taken consistently for an extended time, and is probably the most worrisome side effect associated with this vitamin. Other severe side effects of nicotinic acid are difficulty metabolizing blood sugar (glucose), disturbed heart rhythms, rash over large areas of the skin, and gouty arthritis.

The intestinal side effects of nicotinamide are less severe, and it does not cause the flushing reaction.

Interactions

Nicotinic acid interacts with clonidine used for hypertension and with certain blood and urine tests. See Part IV, "Vitamin, Mineral, and Drug Interactions."

Therapeutic Uses

Niacin supplements may be given to counteract any of the symptoms of niacin deficiency reviewed earlier in this profile. However, such symptoms will not be alleviated by niacin use unless they are, in fact, caused by vitamin deficiency.

In addition to the prevention and cure of the deficiency disease, pellagra, it has been known for a long time that nicotinic acid, when given in megadoses, is capable of reducing levels of the blood fats triglycerides and cholesterol in the blood and has been widely prescribed for this purpose. However, claims that taking niacin for this purpose will increase the life span of patients with heart and blood vessel diseases are unproven—as discussed below.

Interestingly, nicotinamide, the biological equivalent to nicotinic acid as a vitamin, does not have the same ability to lower the levels of these blood lipids.

Unsubstantiated Claims

Prevention of Heart Attacks

In the mid-1960s, the National Heart and Lung Institute funded a coronary drug project involving more than eight thousand patients at fifty-three different clinical centers. Volunteers received long-term treatment with either nicotinic acid, another lipid-lowering agent, or a placebo (inactive drug). Those taking nicotinic acid were given 3 g. (3,000 mg.) each day, almost 190 times the average adult RDA.

The results of this study, one of the most comprehensive

evaluations ever undertaken, showed no evidence that nicotinic acid prolonged the lives of patients who had suffered a heart attack. Although nicotinic acid was clearly responsible for lowering blood levels of cholesterol and triglycerides, the five-year total death rate in both treatment and placebo groups was not significantly different. The niacin group did have a slightly lower incidence of nonfatal heart attacks while they were taking the vitamin, but they also experienced a significant number of serious adverse reactions to their treatment.

Some of these adverse reactions were: disturbances of heart rhythm (arrhythmias), stomach and intestinal problems, liver toxicity, some difficulty handling large amounts of sugar in the blood (diabetic tendency), skin rash, itching, and gouty arthritis. We cannot recommend the routine use of nicotinic acid to prevent heart attack because the vitamin did not affect the overall death rate and may lead to significant adverse reactions.

Alleviation of Mental Illness

A second megavitamin use of nicotinic acid is for mental illnesses, notably schizophrenia, for which it was first used in the early 1950s. The origin of this use came, of course, from the fact that niacin alleviated symptoms of mental illness when they were caused by nicotinic acid deficiency. Some psychiatrists, however, still routinely prescribe daily doses up to 20 g. and hardly a month passes without the appearance of another article extolling the virtues of nicotinic acid and other miracle nutrients in the alleviation of mental illness.

Unfortunately, nicotinic acid has been tested and found ineffective in the treatment of schizophrenia. The most comprehensive of these evaluations was conducted during 1971 by the Canadian Mental Health Association. Their studies were set up as a controlled multicenter evaluation, similar to that described for the evaluation of nicotinic acid for heart disease. The findings of these careful studies are best summarized by saying that the claims of megavitamin enthusiasts have not been confirmed. In a comparison of such factors as the length of hospitalization and the quantity of tranquilizers consumed, the niacin group fared worse than the placebo group.

More recently, Linus Pauling and others have advocated treatment for mental illness known as "orthomolecular psychiatry,'' meaning psychiatric treatment using nutritional agents. Nicotinic acid is a component of this form of treatment, but therapists have added other vitamins, notably C, to their regimens along with strict adherence to a sugar- and food additive-free diet. These complex regimens have not been the subject of scientific scrutiny. Therefore, we cannot advocate their use.

In this context, we would also like to add a comment concerning the concept of mind over matter. Nicotinic acid causes flushing of the face and a tingling sensation which contributes to the impression that the drug is having profound effects on the body. Using these symptoms a compassionate and enthusiastic therapist can improve the well-being of a patient, even though the vitamin does not exert a specific therapeutic effect.

It is attractive to many patients to think that they can circumvent traditional medical therapies and take psychiatric treatment into their own hands. But we believe that using nicotinic acid without other medicines and/or psychotherapy can be both costly and dangerous.

Nicotinic acid has also been promoted for other uses for which its value has not been proven. We cannot recommend that you take this vitamin to treat bad breath, canker sores, deafness, dizziness, depression, hypertension, skin blemishes, or tiredness. Nicotinic acid also will not prevent migraine headaches or senility, nor will it improve digestion.

Availability

Nicotinic acid (niacin) is available in tablets of 25 mg., 50 mg., 100 mg., and 500 mg. Timed-release capsules in similar strengths are also available as is an elixir with 50 mg. in every teaspoonful. These high doses are used to lower blood fat levels as discussed above. Nicotinamide is available in capsules and tablets containing 25 mg., 50 mg., 100 mg., and 500 mg. Larger dosage units of nicotinic acid and vitamin injection are mostly restricted to prescription-only use.

Vitamin B₅
Pantothenic Acid

The name of this vitamin, derived from the word *pan* (Greek for ''all''), means ''from everywhere.'' Pantothenic acid does, indeed, live up to its name; it is found in all living things throughout our environment. As a result, this vitamin is unique in that severe deficiencies in man have never occurred naturally. Symptoms of deficiency have only been produced under experimental conditions.

One of the more intriguing findings about pantothenic acid is the fact that this vitamin reverses the graying process in the hair of black rats. Unfortunately, the graying of rat hair has no relation to the graying of human hair, so this attribute won't help us.

Function

Pantothenic acid is converted in the human body to a catalyst called coenzyme A. Coenzyme A is a high energy compound used in the transfer of a variety of substances during normal body processes. These include the metabolism of carbohydrates, the breakdown of fatty acids, the generation of glucose from glycogen—the form in which it is stored in the liver—and the body processes that make such substances as steroid hormones.

Daily Requirements

There are no established standards for pantothenic acid intake, and it is therefore not included in the RDA tables. However, the Food and Nutrition Board of the National Academy of Sciences has established 4–7 mg. as safe and adequate for daily intake. These standards are only a guess as to daily requirement and cannot be taken as definite needs.

Dietary Sources

Most Western diets contain amounts of pantothenic acid that are more than adequate. Some of the richest sources are corn,

Vitamin B₅ (Pantothenic Acid) Content of Selected Foods

Average adult safe and adequate daily intake is 5.5 mg.

Food	Approximate Content (mg. per 3 oz.)
Almonds	0.43
Apricot nectar	0.86
Avocado	0.94
Beans	0.34
Blue Cheese	1.53
Brewer's yeast	9.35*
Broccoli	0.43
Cashew nuts	1.11
Cheese	0.43
Chicken	0.77
Chickpeas	1.02
Corn	4.25
Eggs	1.96
Egg yolk	3.57
Lamb	0.50
Lentils	4.08
Lobster	1.28
Milk	0.34
Mushrooms	0.85
Peanuts	2.38
Peas	2.90
Pomegranate	0.54
Potatoes	0.50
Salmon	0.68
Sardines	0.77
Soybeans	4.42
Sunflower seeds	4.25
Tuna	0.43
Turkey	0.77
Walnuts	0.77
Wheat germ	1.87*

*Equivalent to 18 teaspoons.

lentils, eggs, nuts, and lobster. Additional good sources are listed on the accompanying table.

Cooking losses of up to 30 percent occur during prolonged heating of foods. Also, much of the pantothenic acid content of whole wheat flour is lost during processing to white flour.

Deficiencies

Under experimental conditions, volunteers fed a pantothenic acid-free diet took ten weeks to develop deficiency symptoms. Others, fed a similar diet and given a substance that counteracts the effects of pantothenic acid, developed the symptoms in a shorter period of time.

Symptoms of Deficiency

The symptoms seen in both of the above groups consisted of nausea, numbness in the extremities, sleep disturbances, muscle spasms and cramps, poor muscle coordination, headache, fatigue, stomach pains, some stomach gas and diarrhea, and occasional vomiting. Subsequent studies have shown that people deprived of pantothenic acid had fewer antibodies in their blood and were not as well protected against foreign substances, such as bacteria.

Prisoners of war during World War II complained of "burning feet" syndrome, associated with tingling and numbness in the legs. These symptoms can occur in anyone who is malnourished and may represent a form of pantothenic acid deficiency, since they respond to vitamin treatment. However, a direct relationship has not been established.

The relationship between symptoms of pantothenic acid deficiency and its function is not always as apparent as that relationship is in other vitamins. However, it is known that a deficiency of pantothenic acid can lead to nerve and muscle disorders because of its role in fat and glucose metabolism, decreased immune response because of an interference with steroid metabolism, and gastrointestinal problems because of an interference with normal cell function in the gastrointestinal tract.

There are no biological tests specific to pantothenic acid deficiency.

Toxicity

Pantothenic acid is nontoxic. People have taken doses as large as 10 g. (10,000 mg.) per day without any known adverse effects.

Therapeutic Uses

Pantothenic acid supplements may be given to counteract the symptoms of pantothenic acid deficiency reviewed earlier in this profile. However, such symptoms will not be alleviated by pantothenic acid unless they are, in fact, caused by vitamin deficiency.

Pantothenic acid is also sold as dexpanthenol (Panthoderm), a lotion or cream to be applied to burns, cuts, or abrasions. This product relieves itching and is soothing to the wound.

Unsubstantiated Claims

Healing

Manufacturers of Panthoderm claim that the product may stimulate wound healing by speeding the formation of new skin, but the claim has not been conclusively proven.

Alleviation of Stress

In recent years, pantothenic acid has been ballyhooed as an "antistress" vitamin. The origins of this alleged property lie in animal studies and the human experiments described under "Deficiencies" above. Advocates of this use of pantothenic acid feel that it will prevent stress and stress-related diseases because people in whom a vitamin deficiency was created were less able to respond to stressful situations. There is, however, no factual evidence that pantothenic acid will prevent or treat any other forms of stress.

Pantothenic acid has also been promoted for other uses for which its value has not yet been proven. We cannot recommend that you take this vitamin to treat alcoholism, allergies, arthritis, constipation, fatigue, liver cirrhosis, shock, or stomach ulcers.

Availability

Pantothenic acid is available without a prescription as calcium pantothenate. It comes in strengths from 10 mg. to 218 mg. Pantothenic acid is also marketed as a lotion or cream under the trade name Panthoderm.

Vitamin B$_6$
Pyridoxine

Vitamin B$_6$ actually consists of three substances—pyridoxine, pyridoxal phosphate, and pyridoxamine—but only pyridoxine is officially designated as B$_6$. All three have equivalent vitamin potency, and the latter two can be utilized by the human body in place of pyridoxine.

Although a great deal is known about the energy-creating processes in which pyridoxine is involved, there are still many unanswered questions about the importance and function of this vitamin in humans. New information is frequently published about pyridoxine, as, for example, the discovery in 1983 of evidence of its toxic potential.

A lack of pyridoxine manifests itself most obviously in the form of nervous system ailments, including seizures.

Function

Pyridoxal phosphate is the active form of vitamin B$_6$ in humans and is manufactured by our bodies from pyridoxine. Magnesium, a nutrient mineral, plays an essential role in phosphate transfer reactions, and people who are magnesium deficient may therefore be less able to make the active form of this vitamin.

Pyridoxal phosphate is required by at least fifty different enzymes, including those involved in the formation of amino acids used as building blocks for protein.

Pyridoxal phosphate is necessary for proper brain and central nervous system function because many chemical transmitters

117

or signals used by the brain for communication depend on B_6 as coenzymes (catalysts) in their formation. Levels of B_6 that are too high, or too low, can affect mental health.

Other important functions of this vitamin include the manufacture of hemoglobin (responsible for carrying oxygen from the lungs to every cell in the body), conversion of carbohydrates into energy, and conversion of the chemical tryptophan to nicotinic acid (vitamin B_3). The latter is essential to normal body operation because about half of our nicotinic acid comes from tryptophan converted by the body.

Daily Requirements

Daily requirements of pyridoxine vary with the amount of protein in the diet. The current recommendation is 1.5 mg. for every 100 g. of dietary protein. The more protein you eat, the greater your need for pyridoxine.

Dietary Sources

In vegetables, B_6 is found as pyridoxine, while in animals and animal products, B_6 activity is supplied by pyridoxal phosphate or pyridoxamine.

The vitamin is present in a variety of foods, and rich sources include meats, grains, fish, eggs, and carrots. Additional good sources are listed in the accompanying table.

There is no evidence to support the contention for widespread B_6 deficiency in the United States, since it can be found in so many foods and some usable B_6 is made by bacteria in the gastrointestinal tract. Routine B_6 supplementation is not necessary, yet it is included in virtually every available multivitamin product.

Pyridoxine is relatively stable in processing, although as much as 25 percent of vitamin activity may be lost during cooking. It is also quite stable when food is frozen or dehydrated, but is destroyed by ultraviolet light and should be stored in dark or opaque containers.

The milling and refining of whole wheat destroys most of its pyridoxine content, which is *not* replaced in the enriched flour used by most consumers.

Vitamin B$_6$ (Pyridoxine) Content of Selected Foods

Average adult RDA is 2 mg.

Food	Approximate Content (mg. per 3 oz.)
Avocado	0.54
Banana	0.51
Beef	0.36
Bran	0.77
Brewer's yeast	3.40*
Carrots	0.59
Cashew nuts	0.36
Eggs	0.43
Fish	0.43
Hazelnuts	1.00
Lentils	1.53
Calves liver	0.60
Peanuts	0.36
Pork	0.28
Potatoes	0.17
Rice	3.24
Salmon	0.88
Soybeans	1.80
Shrimp	0.54
Sunflower seeds	3.24
Tuna	0.81
Turkey	0.36
Wheat germ	0.82
Whole wheat flour	0.51

*Equivalent to 18 teaspoons.

Deficiencies

Since pyridoxine is involved with the functioning of the brain, the formation of hemoglobin in red blood cells, and the manufacture of body proteins, deficiency is reflected by impairment of all these biological functions. While severe pyridoxine deficiency is rarely seen, marginal deficiency may be found in some special circumstances including people taking drugs that interact with pyridoxine. Obvious deficiency states have been produced under test situations by feeding volunteers 4-deoxy-pyridoxine, which counteracts vitamin B_6.

Symptoms of Deficiency

Under test conditions, nervous system abnormalities such as irritability, confusion, nervousness, and numbness of the extremities were observed. Skin lesions similar to those seen with riboflavin (vitamin B_2) and a magenta coloration of the tongue have also resulted after several weeks of a pyridoxine-deficient diet plus the vitamin antagonist 4-deoxypyridoxine. Convulsive seizures can develop if the vitamin is withheld for extended periods. Some time ago, an incident occurred in which three hundred infants were mistakenly given pyridoxine-deficient formula. These children became nervous, and several of them experienced convulsions before the problem was discovered and corrected.

Severe pyridoxine deficiency will cause an anemia in man, but this rarely occurs in people who are simply deficient in dietary pyridoxine intake. When such anemia does develop, it can be easily reversed by simply taking supplemental B_6.

It is possible to determine vitamin B_6 deficiency by giving a person a loading dose (a large dose all at once) of the chemical tryptophan by mouth. The patient will then pass a number of unusual metabolites of tryptophan out of his or her body via the urine. One of these, xanthurenic acid, is a convenient measure of B_6 deficiency. This test, however, is not routinely used.

Pyridoxine and Pregnant Women

Pregnant women need extra pyridoxine for several reasons. The growing fetus requires a considerable amount of energy, extra vitamins, and other nutrients from the mother. Also, estrogenic hormones present in larger than usual amounts during the term of pregnancy tend to change amino acid metabolism and increase the need for pyridoxine. Since abnormally low pyridoxine levels have been reported during pregnancy, expectant mothers should take a special prenatal vitamin formulation that provides about 2.5 mg. of pyridoxine per pill.

Toxicity

B$_6$ is considered to be nontoxic in daily doses up to about 100 mg. But people taking 200 mg. or more per day for a month can become dependent on the vitamin, and some have actually experienced physical symptoms of B$_6$ deficiency when their vitamin was abruptly stopped. Such large daily doses of pyridoxine must be reduced gradually until they are below 100 mg. per day. A reasonable reduction schedule will decrease the dose by about 20 percent every three to five days. Then the vitamin can be stopped without worry.

High doses of B$_6$ cause convulsions in animals. Until recently, there had been no human counterpart to these reports in lab animals. A 1983 report published in the *New England Journal of Medicine* described seven people who suffered severe nerve disorders after taking megadoses of vitamin B$_6$. The doses taken ranged up to 6 g. (6,000 mg.) per day, or 3,000 times the average adult RDA. These people had difficulty walking, their hands became numb and difficult to control, they lost some sensory perception (touch, temperature, vibration, pin prick, and feeling of position), and lost feeling in the area around their mouths. All seven improved after they stopped taking the vitamin, but the recovery took as long as seven months, and some symptoms remained even at that time. Since then, these symptoms have been noted in people taking as little as 500 mg. a day of the vitamin.

Animal studies have shown doses equivalent to 200–600 mg. per day in humans will decrease blood levels of prolactin, a hormone involved in the process of breast milk production. Some people have suggested that B$_6$ be avoided by breastfeeding mothers, but there is no evidence that the amounts of pyridoxine contained in normal vitamin supplements can affect breast milk production.

Interactions

Pyridoxine can interact with barbiturates, levodopa (1-dopa) given for Parkinson's disease, phenytoin for seizures, isoniazid and cycloserine for tuberculosis, hydralazine for hypertension, penicillanime for arthritis and Wilson's disease, oral contraceptives, and vitamin B_{12}. See Part IV, "Vitamin, Mineral, and Drug Interactions," for details.

Therapeutic Uses

Pyridoxine supplements may be given to counteract any symptoms of vitamin B_6 deficiency reviewed earlier in this profile. However, such symptoms will not be alleviated by pyridoxine unless they are, in fact, caused by vitamin deficiency.

In addition, pyridoxine has been found to have some therapeutic value for the following conditions.

Depression Associated with Oral Contraceptives

Preliminary information suggests that supplemental pyridoxine may be of value in partially reversing the depression commonly associated with the use of oral contraceptives (the pill). The reason for this is that the estrogenic component of the pill alters blood levels of pyridoxine and therefore increases daily requirement.

Large-scale controlled trials must be conducted to confirm this important observation. However, we would recommend B_6 supplementation in doses of 25–100 mg. per day to those women taking oral contraceptives who have experienced troublesome depression and not achieved relief from other therapy. Since the depression under consideration here is specifically due to pyridoxine deficiency, vitamin B_6 therapy should not be viewed as generally valuable in the treatment of any other form of depression.

Premenstrual Syndrome

Pyridoxine has also received a lot of publicity as a treatment for this common problem. The theory here is that the symptoms of premenstrual syndrome are caused by a hormone imbalance associated with menstruation. Advocates of this therapy say that the situation is similar to oral contraceptive depression and the marginal deficiencies reported among pregnant women. The problem with this thinking is that both situations can be related to potential aberrations in pyridoxine metabolism lasting longer than a few days a month. There are no data to support this theory, but women suffering from the symptoms of premenstrual tension may want to take a daily multivitamin containing vitamin

B$_6$. It is probably more important to maintain adequate levels of the vitamin and avoid marginal deficiency than to take it only for a few days each month.

Reduction of Breast Milk

Some European physicians have employed daily doses of 50 mg. of pyridoxine to purposely suppress prolactin secretion and reduce milk production in women who have just given birth. High-dose pyridoxine has been hailed as a savior because it may replace the hormones that have been used for this purpose. Only time will tell.

Treating Inborn Errors of Metabolism

There are at least six rare, inherited genetic defects that can be treated by giving high doses of vitamin B$_6$. Studies have shown that, in most cases, these defects are the result of a genetic error that results in the manufacture of a defective enzyme. The defect is usually related to the enzyme's inability to bind tightly to its needed vitamin. If the enzyme cannot bind to the vitamin, it cannot function. Extraordinarily high vitamin doses may be able to "flood" the enzyme so that, even though the vitamin is not tightly bound to the enzyme, it can still work.

These are not true vitamin deficiency diseases. They are defects in a single enzyme that can be overcome by megadoses of the appropriate vitamin. The abnormally low enzyme activity can lead to a variety of symptoms, but usually the problem is revealed during early childhood in the form of mental retardation and failure to grow and thrive.

The following list contains several examples of B$_6$-dependent inborn errors of metabolism. These rare, but serious defects often respond miraculously to vitamin treatment. It must be emphasized that most cases of mental retardation or developmental problems will *not* respond to vitamin treatments. Only a mental retardation specialist can pinpoint those cases which will respond and the exact vitamin needed.

Examples of B$_6$-Dependent Inborn Errors of Metabolism

Name	Symptoms	Amount of B$_6$ Required	Problem
B$_6$-dependent convulsions	Seizures	10–25 mg./day	Defective glutamic acid that results in GABA depletion
Xanthurenic acidurea	Mental retardation	5–10 mg./day	Defective tryptophan metabolism; high levels of xanthurenic acid found in the urine
Cystathionurea	Mental retardation	25–500 mg./day	Defective cystathionase; high cystathionase levels in the urine

Carpal Tunnel Defect

A nerve defect in the wrist called carpal tunnel defect causes loss of strength in the hands and fingers. For an as yet unknown reason, vitamin B$_6$ helps some people with this problem. Perhaps, this is simply another expression of pyridoxine deficiency! Vitamin therapy may be worth a try since the only sure cure is a delicate operation that must be performed by a specialist in orthopedic surgery. Doses of pyridoxine used in one of the more successful studies of carpal tunnel defect were 100 mg. three times a day. We suggest that people desiring pyridoxine therapy for this nerve disorder work with their doctor.

Unsubstantiated Claims

Relief of Morning Sickness

Pyridoxine has been combined with an antihistamine and promoted for the treatment of morning sickness. The product involved was called Benedectin and was used in the United States for almost two decades until it was withdrawn during 1982. The withdrawal was a voluntary action on the part of the manufacturer because of a question as to the potential for this product to cause birth defects: high doses of pyridoxine have caused birth defects in laboratory animals. This data cannot be directly related to human beings, but the drug was withdrawn because of the manufacturer's desire to avoid adverse publicity and the possibility of staggering lawsuits. Thus, the issue was never resolved to anyone's satisfaction.

There has never been any solid evidence to support the role of pyridoxine for morning sickness. Therefore, we would recommend that pregnant or breastfeeding women take pyridoxine only for nutritional purposes. In addition, we would like to stress that there is certainly nothing that would indicate that this vitamin is of value in treating nausea and vomiting caused by conditions other than pregnancy.

Pyridoxine has also been promoted for other uses for which its value has not been proven. We cannot recommend that you take this vitamin to treat arthritis, diabetes, mental retardation, numbness, or obesity. Pyridoxine will also not prevent aging, fluid retention, or leg cramp, nor can it improve your vision or help you lose weight.

Availability

Vitamin B_6, as pyridoxine hydrochloride tablets, can be purchased without a prescription in strengths between 5 and 500 mg. Several timed-release preparations are also available, but the value of timed-release vitamins (except nicotinic acid) is questionable. Pyridoxine hydrochloride (50 and 100 mg.) injection is available only on a doctor's prescription.

Vitamin B_{12}
Cyanocobolamine

Unlike the other B vitamins, B_{12} is not produced by plants—the major producers of B_{12} are the bacteria in our environment. Animal species feed on these bacteria and pick up the B_{12} to pass along the food chain. Therefore, understanding of the role of this vitamin is particularly important for partial vegetarians and vegans.

The inability of some people to absorb vitamin B_{12} causes Addison's disease, or pernicious anemia, a life-threatening disease demanding immediate and vigorous treatment. B_{12} was discovered in 1948 and first used to treat pernicious anemia in dogs.

Compared with the other vitamins, B_{12} is a very large molecule, with a weight of 1355; nicotinic acid, for instance, has a molecular weight of only 123. Cobolamine, which contains the trace mineral cobalt, is the pure form of this vitamin. However, the common available form of B_{12}, cyanocobolamine, is not found in nature, but was accidentally discovered by a pharmaceutical researcher attempting to purify cobolamine. Cyanocobolamine is the most convenient way for people to supplement their B_{12} intake because of its stability. However, hydroxycobolamine, the chemical precursor to cyanocobolamine, offers some advantages to people with a documented B_{12} deficiency. It is absorbed more slowly after injection into a muscle than cyanocobolamine and is stored in larger quantities by the liver. Hydroxycobolamine produces a more sustained rise in B_{12} levels and a slower elimination of the vitamin from the body. For these reasons, hydroxycobolamine is preferable to cyanocobolamine and should be used whenever possible.

function

Vitamin B_{12} acts in concert with folic acid in reactions that are critical to the process of normal cell division and are required for the synthesis of DNA and RNA, the architects of every cell and function in the body. Body tissue cannot divide and grow normally without vitamin B_{12}, and its role is particularly vital in the area of bone marrow tissue, where blood cells are manufactured.

B_{12} also participates in the regeneration of folic acid by body enzymes. Without B_{12}, we would not be able to reuse the folic acid in our bodies and would require massive amounts of that vitamin. It is unlikely that we would be able routinely to supply enough folic acid from our diets on a continuous basis to support life.

Another important function of B$_{12}$ is its essential role in the metabolism of body fats. The body has a strange way of handling the many fats that contain odd numbers of carbon atoms. Normally, fats with an even number of carbons are chopped into neat little two-carbon units, which are then fed directly into our main energy-producing mechanisms, the glycolysis and tricarboxylic acid cycles. Fats that have an odd number of carbon atoms in them are chopped up in the same way as even-numbered lipids until the process is almost completed. B$_{12}$ facilitates the breakdown of the final three-carbon unit.

Cobolamine appears to be important in two other ways as well. The first involves maintaining sulfhydryl compounds in a reduced state. This is important because reduced sulfhydryl prevents the addition of excessive amounts of oxygen to some fats and other compounds. Oxygen is necessary because it is employed in certain body reactions that release energy, but too much oxygen will lead to destruction of body tissue. Secondly, B$_{12}$, through its role in fat metabolism, participates in the manufacture of a material called myelin, which sheathes and protects nerve fibers. People who are deficient in B$_{12}$ will produce faulty myelin and can, if the deficiency lasts long enough, develop damage to some peripheral nerves and portions of the spinal cord.

Daily Requirements

The average adult RDA for B$_{12}$ is 3 mcg., and most people do not require supplemental B$_{12}$ for any reason.

This vitamin is an exception to the axiom that water-soluble vitamins are not stored in the body in large quantities for extended periods of time. The liver has an extremely efficient storage mechanism to retain B$_{12}$ and usually holds about a thousand-day supply. Even if you were to stop taking in B$_{12}$ completely, it would take from three to five years for deficiency symptoms to develop. A functioning intestinal absorption system for B$_{12}$ is a must, of course, because some of your B$_{12}$ passes into the gastrointestinal tract via the bile after it has been used and is then reabsorbed.

Dietary Sources

Most of us receive B_{12} as cobolamine derivatives found in fish and shellfish, beef, and dairy products (also from animals), though a little may be found in legumes—plants that have a special relationship with certain soil bacteria. Liver, clams, and sardines

Vitamin B_{12} (Cyanocobolamine) Content of Selected Foods
Average adult RDA is 3 mcg.

Food	Approximate Content (mcg. per 3 oz.)
Bass	1.10
Beef	1.70
Blue Cheese	1.20
Camembert cheese	1.00
Chicken	0.43
Clam broth	8.50
Clams	17.00
Crab	0.72
Eggs	1.70
Flounder	5.10
Gorgonzola cheese	1.00
Halibut	1.10
Herring	8.50
Liver	77.40
Liverwurst	1.20
Lobster	1.10
Mackerel	8.50
Milk	0.34
Pork	0.51
Sardines	29.00
Sausage	0.94
Scallops	0.70
Shrimp	0.70
Snapper	7.50
Swiss cheese	1.70
Turkey	0.36

are by far the richest sources, but cheeses that are rich in bacteria, such as Camembert and Gorgonzola, are also good. Additional good sources are listed in the accompanying table.

Since B$_{12}$ is stored in liver and, to a lesser extent, in muscle tissue, people who get some of their calories from meat receive ample amounts of dietary B$_{12}$ (5–15 mcg. per day in the normal Western diet).

Foods containing vitamin B$_{12}$ should be protected from light but are relatively stable; less than 30 percent of B$_{12}$ content is lost during cooking.

Deficiencies

The classic B$_{12}$ deficiency disease, pernicious anemia, does not often develop because of inadequate amounts of the vitamin in the diet. It is usually related to a problem in absorbing the vitamin from the small intestine into the bloodstream. This complex process requires hydrochloric acid and a compound simply known as intrinsic factor. Intrinsic factor is a complex protein made by special cells in the stomach lining that facilitate the absorption of vitamin B$_{12}$.

Symptoms of Deficiency

The symptoms of pernicious anemia include a gradual, and possibly permanent, loss of reflexes, nerve sensation, and function due to the production of faulty myelin sheaths, which may or may not return after treatment with B$_{12}$. This damage is often felt as tingling and numbness in the arms and legs, unusual mood swings, memory losses, or visual difficulties, but can show up in a variety of other forms, depending on the nerve or nerves damaged.

The actual diagnosis of pernicious anemia must be made by a doctor based on the analysis of your blood. Typically, he will find an unusually large proportion of immature or abnormal red blood cells because they cannot proceed through the stages of normal maturation.

The concentration of B$_{12}$ in the blood can be measured directly. Tests for pernicious anemia also include tests of stomach function, to make sure that you have enough hydrochloric acid, and the Schilling test, a test that measures your ability to absorb what B$_{12}$ is available in your diet.

129

Other deficiency symptoms are those caused by megaloblastic anemia, which is usually associated with folic acid deficiency (p. 137) but can occur here because of the close working relationship between B_{12} and folic acid. The symptoms include irritability, weakness, lack of energy, sleeping difficulties, and loss of facial color.

Vitamin B₁₂ and Vegetarians

A vegetarian who consumes milk, other dairy products, or eggs will receive adequate amounts of B_{12}. The vegan (one who avoids all animal-derived foods), though, will usually get little B_{12} in his or her diet. In actual practice B_{12} deficiency is not that common among vegetarians, as a group.

We suggest that strict vegetarians take a regular B_{12} supplement to be on the safe side. This is most inexpensively and conveniently accomplished by purchasing a multivitamin that contains B_{12}. Vegetarians can rest assured that supplemental B_{12} is not obtained from animal products; it is prepared commercially as a by-product of the fermentation processes used in making some antibiotics.

Vitamin B₁₂ and Other Special Groups

Other categories of people who are likely to need B_{12} supplement are pregnant or breastfeeding women (4 mcg. a day is recommended) and senior citizens who may not be getting proper nutrition. Some experts have suggested that seniors who develop psychosis should be evaluated for their B_{12} status before other treatments are given.

Additional B_{12} may also be needed by people with severe illnesses who must be sure that they have enough B_{12} to allow active tissue growth and healing and those who have had their stomachs surgically removed.

Toxicity

Vitamin B_{12} is generally considered nontoxic.

Interactions

Vitamin B_{12} can interact with animmnosalicylic acid (PAS) used for tuberculosis, colcicine used for gout, the antibiotic chloramphenicol (Chloromycetin) and neomycin, vitamin B$_6$, and vitamin C. See Part IV, "Vitamin, Mineral, and Drug Interactions."

Therapeutic Uses

The only recognized therapeutic use for vitamin B$_{12}$ is to prevent and correct pernicious anemia. It should be noted here that once B$_{12}$ has been given to correct pernicious anemia, the treatment must be continued for life to bypass faulty vitamin absorption mechanisms.

We strongly discourage the use of "shotgun" antianemia therapies that combine a number of factors (iron, B$_{12}$, folate, etc.) often used in treating anemia, unless prescribed by a doctor. The use of folate-containing preparations can hide the obvious symptoms of B$_{12}$ deficiency.

Unsubstantiated Claims

Cure for Lack of Energy

It has been the unfortunate practice of many physicians to administer monthly B$_{12}$ injections for tiredness, undiagnosed anemia, and other vague symptoms. The dose usually given is 1,000 mcg., ten times the usually recommended injectable dose and about six months' worth of B$_{12}$, in terms of the usual daily rate. This practice is costly, unnecessary, and potentially dangerous because it exposes the patient to the possibility of reactions to the injection. Allergic reactions to B$_{12}$ injection can involve itching, redness, swelling, and, in rare cases, serious drug reactions. If supplements are needed and your intestinal absorption mechanism is intact, take B$_{12}$ by mouth in liquid or pill form.

Vitamin B$_{12}$ has also been promoted for other uses for which its value has not been proven. B$_{12}$ also will not improve resistance to infection and disease, increase appetite, or promote growth; nor will it improve memory or the ability to learn.

Availability

Vitamin B$_{12}$ is available without a prescription as cyanocobalamine tablets in strengths from 10 to 250 mcg. It is also available on prescription in dosage strengths of 500–1,000 mcg.

Cyanocobolamine injections are available in strengths ranging from 30 to 1,000 mcg./ml., but they require a doctor's prescription. Hydroxycobolamine also requires a prescription and is available only as an injection (1,000 mcg./ml.). Most multivitamins that contain B_{12} have about 6 mcg. per tablet.

Vitamin H
Biotin

Though it is one of the less-publicized vitamins, biotin actually plays an important role in the metabolism of carbohydrates and fats.

Deficiencies of this vitamin are extremely rare in man because biotin is found in almost all living things and is made in our own gastrointestinal tract by microorganisms that are normally present. The only known way to develop a biotin deficiency is to eat large quantities of raw egg whites because they contain a substance called Avidin which prevents biotin from being absorbed into the blood. Symptoms of this deficiency are therefore collectively called egg white injury.

Function

Biotin serves as a catalyst in the chemical reaction—called carbon dioxide fixation—that attaches carbon dioxide to other molecules. The first step in carbon dioxide fixation is binding to biotin; then the carbon dioxide molecule is attached to the appropriate acceptor muscle. The role that biotin plays in the process makes it an important ingredient in the metabolism of carbohydrate (sugar) and fat.

Daily Requirements

The Food and Nutrition Board of the National Academy of Sciences has determined that 100–200 mcg. per day are estimated a safe and adequate level for daily intake among adults. Infants require only 35–50 mcg. per day.

Dietary Sources

Rich dietary sources of biotin include liver, soybeans, sunflower seeds, butter, eggs, nuts, and several vegetables. Additional good sources are listed in the accompanying table. Biotin is stable in normal food processing and cooking.

Vitamin H (Biotin) Content of Selected Foods

The estimated safe and adequate daily intake is 150 mcg.

Food	Approximate Content (mcg. per 3 oz.)
Almonds	15.0
Beans	14.5
Bran	12.0
Brewer's yeast*	170.0
Butter	85.0
Cashew nuts	25.5
Cauliflower	15.0
Chickpeas	27.2
Clams	17.0
Eggs	17.0
Green peas	36.0
Lentils	36.0
Calf's liver	102.0
Mackerel	17.0
Mushrooms	13.6
Peanuts	34.0
Pecans	25.5
Rice	60.0
Salmon	13.0
Sardines	20.0
Soybeans	161.5
Split peas	70.0
Sunflower seeds	60.0
Tuna	25.5
Walnuts	34.0

*Equivalent to 18 teaspoons.

Deficiencies

Natural biotin deficiency is almost unheard of in man. However, deficiency symptoms have been found in a small number of people whose total nutritional requirements were being provided by intravenous feeding. Biotin deficiency has also been produced by feeding volunteers large numbers of raw eggs.

Symptoms of Deficiency

Symptoms noted among test volunteers were nausea, loss of appetite, numbness, muscle pains, rashes, depression, anemia, and high blood cholesterol.

However, one of the most complete descriptions of biotin deficiency was recently made by doctors in San Francisco. They reported on a woman who developed symptoms of biotin deficiency after surgery to remove a large section of diseased intestine. The woman developed a rash, lost her body hair, had a "waxy" appearance, and was tired all the time. She showed remarkable improvement after only a few weeks of treatment with 10 mg. per day of biotin by injection. All of the deficiency symptoms disappeared after a month of biotin treatment.

A specific kind of infant rash, called seborrheic dermatitis, is probably a form of biotin deficiency and can be cured by giving biotin. The low biotin content of both mother's milk and cow's milk can account for the deficiency in infants, although many obtain sufficient biotin from microorganisms in their intestines. Formula-fed infants do not develop this problem.

A small number of rare inborn errors of metabolism due to biotin deficiency can be cured by giving massive amounts of the vitamin.

There are no direct tests for biotin deficiency.

Toxicity

Biotin is generally nontoxic in humans.

Therapeutic Uses

There are no recognized therapeutic uses for biotin.

Unsubstantiated Claims

Biotin has been promoted for other uses for which its value has not been proven. We cannot recommend that you take this vitamin for baldness or depression.

Availability

Biotin is added to some multivitamin formulations and is also available in tablets of 100 mcg., 300 mcg., and 600 mcg.

Folic Acid

Folic acid is so called because it was first isolated from green leafy vegetables. (Latin *folium* means foliage or leaf.)

Folic acid works closely with vitamin B_{12} and is vital to the creation of healthy red blood cells. Deficiency can lead to a particular form of anemia called megaloblastic anemia, after the technical name for improperly formed blood cells.

The term *folic acid* refers to all compounds with folic acid activity, including the two forms of the vitamin that exist in nature—folate and folacin. All forms of folic acid have equivalent vitamin activity and can be interchanged. Folic acid requirements and food concentrations are expressed as folacin equivalents.

Function

Folic acid acts in concert with vitamin B_{12} in reactions that are critical to the process of normal cell division and are required for the synthesis of RNA and DNA, the architects of every cell and function in the body. At least six active folic acid derivatives are used in this process, which is particularly important in the areas of bone marrow tissue where blood cells are manufactured.

Daily Requirements

In the normal adult, the minimum requirement has been scientifically estimated at 50 mcg. per day, but the average adult

RDA is set at 400 mcg. However, since folic acid is necessary for cell division, it follows that folate needs are increased during periods of injury or illness.

Dietary Sources

Green leafy vegetables are a good source of this vitamin, as its name implies, but liver and many beans and seeds contain even more folic acid. There is relatively little folic acid in fruits and lean meats.

Cow's milk and human milk contain more than enough folic acid to prevent vitamin deficiency in infants, but goat's milk is very low in folate. Infants fed goat's milk will need extra folic acid to prevent deficiency from developing. Additional sources of folic acid are listed in the accompanying table.

Folate (Folacin) Content of Selected Foods
Average adult RDA is 400 mcg.

Food	Approximate Content (mcg. per 3 oz.)
Almonds	42.50
Asparagus	102.00
Bananas	25.50
Barley	179.00
Beans	255.00
Bran	40.00
Brazil nuts	42.50
Brewer's yeast*	1,700.00
Broccoli	42.50
Brussels sprouts	42.50
Cashew nuts	21.25
Chickpeas	349.00
Coconut	25.50
Collard greens	85.00
Corn	51.00
Cottage cheese	25.50
Eggs	25.50
Endive	400.00

Folate (Folacin) Content of Selected Foods

Food	Approximate Content (mcg. per 3 oz.
Greens	51.00
Hazelnuts	60.00
Kale	60.00
Lentils	289.00
Calves liver	247.00
Orange juice	54.00
Peanuts	51.00
Peas	110.00
Pecans	25.50
Rice	145.00
Soybeans	595.00
Spinach	68.00
Split peas	196.00
Sprouts	119.00
Sunflower seeds	85.00
Vegetable greens	51.00
Walnuts	51.00
Wheat	187.00
Wheat germ*	264.00

*Equivalent to 18 teaspoons.

Folic acid is one of the least stable vitamins in cooking and processing, particularly in regard to vegetables and dairy products. It has been estimated that more than 90 percent of folic acid content may be lost from vegetables when they are cooked (so much for cooked spinach!). However, little is lost from meats when they are cooked.

Deficiencies

Since folic acid is essential for cell division and reproduction, organs and tissues that divide rapidly are severely affected by folate deficiency.

Bone marrow, which produces blood cells, is one such

tissue. Folic acid deficiency causes the bone marrow to become less efficient in making new blood cells and produces megaloblastic anemia. The differentiation between megaloblastic and other types of anemia, such as iron deficiency or pernicious anemia, can only be made by your doctor on the basis of information gleaned from laboratory analyses of your blood.

Folate deficiency is also a common complication of diseases of the stomach and intestines that can interfere with the absorption of this vitamin.

Studies have shown that people consuming a folate-deficient diet take between three and five months to show signs of deficiency; as with some other water-soluble vitamins, the body maintains limited stores of folic acid to provide a reserve during periods of low intake.

Symptoms of Deficiency

People with folate deficiency experience many of the same symptoms as those with other forms of anemia: irritability, weakness, lack of energy, sleeping difficulties, and loss of facial color. Unlike B_{12}, nerve damage does not develop.

Folate levels can be measured directly in the blood. Normal concentrations range from 4 to 20 nanograms per milliliter. Anything less than 4 ng./ml. is considered a deficiency. Changes in the process of making red blood cells become apparent within a week or two after the levels of vitamin become deficient, and symptoms may develop anytime thereafter.

Folic Acid and Alcoholics

Alcoholics are often folate deficient because of their vastly restricted food intake and the fact that alcohol interferes with body reactions that prepare folic acid for reuse. Today, alcoholism is the number 1 cause of folic acid deficiency.

Folic Acid and Pregnant Women

Pregnant women need at least 800 mcg. per day because of the rapid rate at which fetal tissues are produced. Breastfeeding women also need this amount because they must supply enough folic acid in their milk to support their baby's rapid growth. Folate deficiency is the most common cause of anemia during pregnancy because more is required and it is relatively difficult to eat foods containing at least 800 mcg. daily. Therefore, we would strongly recommend that pregnant women take a daily prenatal vitamin containing at least 800 mcg. (0.8 mg.) of folic acid.

Drugs and Folic Acid Deficiency

Some prescription drugs can interfere with your absorption of folic acid and thereby lead to deficiencies. These are: methotrexate for cancer, phenytoin for seizures, trimethroprim for infection and triamterene, which is one of the ingredients in the diuretic medication Dyrenium. Supplementation may be needed if anemia develops while taking these medications.

Toxicity

Folic acid is considered to be nontoxic to man; daily doses as large as 15 mg. have been well tolerated. However, large amounts of folic acid may counteract the effects of phenytoin, primidone and phenobarbital, for seizures, antiepileptic medicines, and pyrimethamine and trimethoprim for infection.

Interactions

Folic acid can interact with chloramphenicol (Chloromycetin), an antibiotic, pyrimethamine (Daraprim) for malaria, and phenytoin for seizures. See Part IV "Vitamin, Mineral, and Drug Interactions."

Therapeutic Uses

Folic acid is only effective in treating anemias due to simple folate deficiency. Adequate diagnosis is necessary before you begin treatment because folic acid will mask the symptoms of a more serious vitamin B_{12} deficiency.

One area of recent controversy is whether women taking oral contraceptives (the pill) should be given routine folic acid supplements. The pill can lower folate levels in women who are already deficient in folic acid and result in anemia. Women receiving sufficient amounts of folic acid from their diet will probably not experience this effect.

Until more is known about the role of the pill in folic acid metabolism, vitamins containing small doses of folic acid may be taken to avoid potential problems. This may be especially important for women. But you must avoid taking more than 1 mg. (1,000 mcg.) daily so that you don't interfere with the possible diagnosis of a B_{12} deficiency.

Folic Acid as a Research Drug

Research into the role of folic acid in body metabolism has led to the development of some life-saving drugs. A folic acid inhibitor, methotrexate, has become one of our most important anticancer drugs. This agent has a selective effect on rapidly dividing cancer cells, which, of course, need lots of folate and other nutrients. Knowledge of the folate cycle has led to further sophistication of treatment with methotrexate. Cancer patients, in a procedure known as leucovorin rescue, are given what might ordinarily be lethal doses of methotrexate and then given calcium leucovorin, an intermediate in the folate cycle that bypasses the blockade created by methotrexate. Interestingly, normal cells are rescued by leucovorin before cancer cells.

The bacterial enzyme which converts folic acid to its active form, tetrahydrofolic acid, is different from the enzyme found in man. A selective inhibitor of the bacterial enzyme, trimethoprim, has been developed and is useful as an antibacterial medicine. Trimethoprim is usually prescribed in combination with a sulfa drug, which inhibits the bacteria's ability to make folic acid.

The two agents work together to produce a greater effect than either could if they were used alone. These medications have few side effects because they don't have a major effect on human enzymes that change folic acid to tetrahydrofolic acid. Research will, as time passes, produce even more medicines that exert their effects through the folic acid cycle.

Unsubstantiated Claims

Folic acid has also been promoted for other uses for which its value has not been proven. We cannot recommend that you take this vitamin to treat pain or skin blemishes. Folic acid will also not improve lactation, increase resistance to infection, protect against internal parasites and food poisoning, prevent canker sores, or delay the onset of gray hair.

Availability

Folic acid is sold on prescription only in tablets of 1 mg. each. Folic acid injection is also available only by prescription. Folic acid in strengths of 0.1 mg., 0.4 mg., and 0.8 mg. may be purchased without a prescription. Folic acid is also included as an ingredient of many vitamin combinations, where the same basic rules apply. Vitamins with more than 0.8 mg. of folic acid can be obtained only on prescription. Vitamins containing 0.8 mg. or less of folic acid per tablet or capsule can be bought without a prescription.

Many multivitamin preparations contain no folic acid. Others contain only small amounts of this vitamin because doses of 1 mg. or more per day can mask the symptoms of B_{12} deficiency, pernicious anemia.

Vitamin C
Ascorbic Acid

Despite a long history of experience and research associated with vitamin C—dating back several centuries, to the search for the cause of scurvy among sailors on long voyages—we still have a lot to learn about how it works in the human body. We know that man is one of the few creatures on earth that doesn't make his own vitamin C, but we don't know why.

Linus Pauling and others think that man's inability to make ascorbic acid and the decrease in C content of our diets over the years—particularly as early man shifted from an all vegetarian diet to a partly meat diet—has placed us at risk for taking in less vitamin C than we need to perform everyday functions.

Some advocates of vitamin C are quick to point out that animals which make their own vitamin C produce the human equivalent of 10–20 g. (10,000–20,000 mg.) per day, while the average human diet contains only 30 mg. per day; they also point to the ape, who eats an average of 5 g. of C per day in the wild. This is disputed by many nutritional experts, who claim that man's diet was probably never strictly vegetarian and that he has always eaten both meats and vegetables. Conventional wisdom tells us that if the ability to make vitamin C had been needed by early man, we would be able to make our own today.

Some evidence indicates that animals make their own vitamin C in large amounts because they use it up much faster than we do. But perhaps man is more efficient than most members of the animal kingdom, in that he can store small amounts of the vitamin C taken in. Why carry the machinery to make vitamin C when you can let plants do it for you?

The arguments on either side of this discussion are pure speculation, and no one can conclusively prove any of the points. The only way advocates of megadose vitamin C therapy can convince the skeptics is to show that these large amounts of vitamin C will result in a long-term benefit. As yet, this has not been proven. Vitamin C may be of value in some illnesses, but there is no evidence to support the concept that everyone should take large amounts of ascorbic acid.

Additional basic research must be undertaken to uncover more information about the exact role of this vitamin.

Chemically, vitamin C is simply a modified sugar molecule. Unlike the other water-soluble vitamins, C probably acts directly in the body without being changed.

function

It is known that vitamin C is necessary in the body process that makes a chemical called hydroxyproline. Hydroxyproline is the most important building block of collagen, the main supporting component in the tissues that hold us together, the so-called connective tissues. Some examples of connective tissue are cartilage, tendons, and fibers. Lack of vitamin C directly affects collagen, causing defects in the formation of teeth and bones, interfering with the normal healing of wounds, and causing the smallest blood vessels, the capillaries, to break. The role of collagen in capillary breakage is related to the breakdown of tissue that surrounds and supports the capillaries. When this tissue breaks down because of vitamin C deficiency, the capillaries break from lack of support, resulting in black and blue bruise marks as blood leaks into tissue and clots there. Other biological functions of vitamin C are not as well understood.

Vitamin C also stimulates the adrenal glands to manufacture cortisone and other body hormones involved in helping us cope with the stresses of daily life. And vitamin C is known to participate in the production of the neurohormone epinephrine. Epinephrine is essential to life because it stimulates many nerves in the central nervous system and in all of our major organs. We could not live without epinephrine.

Vitamin C increases the amount of iron from non-meat sources absorbed through the intestines, and it is involved in the conversion of folic acid to its active form, folinic acid, in the body. In fact, one of the features of vitamin C deficiency is an anemia similar to the kind found in people deficient in folic acid. Small amounts of ascorbic acid are also needed to break down cholesterol in the blood.

White blood cells contain relatively large amounts of vitamin C, and its presence seems to be key to the ability of these cells to attack and engulf invading bacteria. In addition, vitamin C is involved in the manufacture of a group of enzymes that are essential to the body's ability to break down drugs and other chemicals the body considers foreign.

Finally, vitamin C may protect body enzymes from unwanted effects of oxygen by tying up the oxygen molecule. This is considered a protective effect because it allows the enzymes to retain their activity. The exact importance of this role is not known since it is not required under ordinary conditions.

Daily Requirements

Some expert estimates indicate that adults require only 10 mg. of ascorbic acid each day to protect against deficiency. Nevertheless, the average adult RDA for ascorbic acid is 60 mg. to replace the amount the body uses and that which is excreted from the body.

Dietary Sources

Fruits, potatoes, and green vegetables are the best natural sources of this vitamin. There is little vitamin C in meats, cereals, grains, and the foods we normally think of as being loaded with B vitamins. Interestingly, the richest sources of vitamin C are not the citrus fruits, as we have been led to believe, but rose hips, broccoli, Brussels sprouts, and green peppers. Additional good sources are listed in the accompanying table.

Vitamin C (Ascorbic Acid) Content of Selected Foods
Average adult RDA is 60 mg.

Food	Approximate Content (mg. per 3 oz.)
Bananas	8.5
Black currants	220.0
Broccoli	110.5
Brussels sprouts	119.0
Cabbage	30.0
Grapefruit	34.0
Green peppers	93.5
Guava	226.0
Calves liver	30.0
Lemons	31.0
Lime	28.0
Oranges	42.5
Orange juice	51.0
Potatoes	21.3
Radishes	21.6
Rose hips	2,550.0
Spinach	76.5
Strawberries	51.3
Tomatoes	21.3
Watercress	72.0

Vitamin C is chemically unstable and therefore presents some problems in terms of storage and processing.

Drying fruits and vegetables destroys much of their vitamin C content. In one experiment, up to 54 percent of the vitamin was destroyed by drying. Vitamin C is also degraded after exposure to light and air. In addition, long storage of fruits and vegetables allows the vitamin to be degraded by enzymes present in that fruit or vegetable.

Another problem unique to ascorbic acid is the time that fruits and vegetables are picked. If picked before they reach their fully ripened state, they will not have produced their full quota of vitamin C.

Freezing does not destroy the vitamin C content of foods. A typical cup of freshly squeezed orange juice contains 100 mg. of ascorbic acid, while a cup of juice prepared from a frozen concentrate and reconstituted contains about 120 mg. of the vitamin, probably because of a special effort to concentrate ascorbic acid during the quick freezing process and the fact that vitamin C is most stable in an acid media, such as fruit juices. However, the vitamin in frozen orange juice can be broken down by oxygen as soon as the juice is reconstituted and warmed to refrigeration temperatures.

Estimates of actual cooking losses range between 10 and 30 percent, although some procedures, such as the combined blanching of vegetables and then cooking them in iron or copper pots can result in the destruction of almost all of the vitamin C.

Deficiencies

The hallmark of vitamin C deficiency is scurvy, the classic disease of sailors in the days before vitamin C was known. Hard hit also were people in northern climates who did not have access to fresh fruits and vegetables during the long winter months.

Our ability to transport fresh food over large distances has dramatically decreased the amount of scurvy worldwide. Nevertheless, marginal vitamin C deficiencies still exist in some people, even in Westernized countries. It takes several months of a vitamin C–deficient diet before scurvy develops. However, marginal deficiencies can develop sooner if you ignore even the most minimal intake of vitamin C.

Symptoms of Deficiency

Our basic descriptions of the symptoms of scurvy come from the logs Jacques Cartier kept during long sea voyages. Cartier's log, written in 1535, graphically tells how severe the disease can be:

The said unknown sickness began to spread itself amongst us at the strangest sort that was ever heard or seen; inasmuch that some did lose all their strength and could not stand upon their feet; then did their legs swell, their sinews shrunk and became black as coal. Others also their skins spotted with spots of blood, of a purple colour. It ascended up their ankles, knees, thighs, shoulders, arms and neck. The mouth became stinking; their gums so rotten that the flesh came away to the roots of their teeth, which at last did fall out.

The latter is, of course, a description of periodontal disease, which can be caused by vitamin C deficiency as well as other factors.

Some symptoms of marginal deficiency are shortness of breath, digestive difficulties, bleeding gums, easy bruisability, swollen or painful bone joints, nosebleeds, anemia (weakness, tiredness, loss of color), more frequent infections, slow wound healing. Some nutrition experts claim that people deficient in C and at risk for heart attacks or strokes are more likely to develop one of these serious problems because of blood vessel weakness.

Vitamin C can be measured directly in the blood. The symptoms of scurvy start to appear when the blood level falls below 1 mg. for every 100 ml. (a little more than 3 oz.) of blood. The vitamin can also be measured in white blood cells. These levels are often taken as a better representation of the amount of vitamin C in body tissues because they are not as subject to variation as the blood level.

Vitamin C and Senior Citizens

Marginal C deficiencies have been reported among seniors, particularly those living in nursing homes or other health care facilities. The reasons for this deficiency seem to be inattention to diet, the loss of appetite, and in some cases, difficulty digesting foods rich in vitamin C, many of which are also high roughage foods. On the basis of this information, we suggest that all people over age sixty-five take a daily multivitamin containing at least 60 mg. of ascorbic acid. Of course, this does not eliminate the need for a balanced diet, including vitamin C rich foods, but it does provide a measure of protection against possible deficiencies.

Vitamin C and Other Special Groups

Pregnant women should supplement their daily vitamin C intake because of the demands placed by developing bones, teeth, and connective tissue. Breastfeeding women also need supplemental C because they must supply enough vitamin C in their milk to support their baby's rapid growth. Smokers, women who take oral contraceptives (the pill), people under any kind of stress, including those with infections, a medical illness, or those experiencing psychological stress, should supplement their daily intake of vitamin C, but the amount does not have to exceed 250 mg. per day.

Toxicity

Considering the vast amounts of vitamin C ingested in the United States, the potential toxicity of doses of 1 g. or more of vitamin C should be of concern. However, recent large-scale clinical trials using over seven thousand volunteers who received between 1 and 30 g. of vitamin C per day revealed very few problems. The long term ingestion of gram quantities of vitamin C has not been carefully studied and we suggest that more doses be used if supplements are designed (less than 250 mg.).

There are scattered reports of a variety of adverse reactions, including stomach upset and diarrhea, but these should be considered rare occurrences. Megadoses, however, can lead to the formation of crystals in the urinary tract and possibly kidney stones. These crystals can interfere with elimination of uric acid and increase the possibility of gout. If you have bladder problems, kidney stones, or gout, you should not use large amounts of vitamin C because of potential problems associated with crystals.

Sudden stoppages of large doses of vitamin C can result in deficiency symptoms, including scurvy. This is also true of infants born of mothers who consume megadoses of vitamin C. They have developed deficiency symptoms soon after birth, probably because their body tissues had become used to very large amounts of vitamin C in the blood circulating from their mother. Infants who develop scurvy immediately after birth have to be given extra vitamin C on a gradually reduced dosage until symptoms have been resolved.

Interactions

Vitamin C can interact with sulfa drugs, aminosalicylic acid (PAS) for tuberculosis, antidepressant drugs, alcohol, oral anticoagulant drugs including warfarin, vitamin B_{12}, iron, calcium, and copper. It can also interfere with certain urine and blood tests. See Part IV, "Vitamin, Mineral, and Drug Interactions."

Therapeutic Uses

Vitamin C supplements may be given to counteract any of the standard symptoms of vitamin C deficiency reviewed earlier in this profile. However, such symptoms will not be alleviated by vitamin C unless they are, in fact, caused by vitamin deficiency.

In addition, vitamin C is often given after surgery to speed healing of the surgical wound. We consider this to be a valid therapeutic use if given in normal, not megadoses, since we know that stress associated with broken bones and other traumatic injuries uses up vitamin C stores in the body faster than normal. Therefore it seems reasonable to expect that extra vitamin C could increase collagen synthesis and thereby enhance the healing process.

A recent, carefully executed study also showed that 600–1,000 mg. per day of ascorbic acid helped people suffering from herpes cold sores get better in half the time. It is not known at this time whether doses smaller than 600 mg. per day would also produce this effect.

Unsubstantiated Claims

Prevention and Cure of the Common Cold

The claim that vitamin C will cure or prevent the common cold is of obvious interest to everyone. This is not a new idea, but was popularized in 1970 with the publication of *Vitamin C and the Common Cold*, by Dr. Linus Pauling. Incredibly, surveys have shown that as many as half the American people have, at some time, taken extra vitamin C to prevent or treat the common cold, an illness responsible for billions of dollars' worth of lost time and productivity each year. Advocates of this treatment claim that 1–10 g. a day of ascorbic acid will prevent the common cold and that higher doses are useful in treating cold symptoms, if you are unlucky enough to get sick in spite of the prevention regimen.

What is the evidence? Vitamin C advocates usually cite the results of studies conducted in the 1940s and 1950s, but most of these early studies are technically incorrect and have been criticized for that reason. The publication of Linus Pauling's book and the increased popularity of vitamin C have sparked careful reevaluations by a number of reputable investigators. At least ten careful, technically correct studies have appeared in the literature since 1970. What emerges from these investigations is a picture far less optimistic than that presented by Linus Pauling and other advocates.

The first study, done in Toronto, Canada, and reported in 1972, indicated that 1 g. of ascorbic acid per day reduced the severity of cold symptoms among university students by about 30 percent, as measured by the number of days lost from work or school because of the cold. There was no significant reduction in the number of colds. This investigation was followed by another, more complex evaluation, reported in 1974, in which the same investigators were unable to duplicate the results of their first study. The reduction in both the number and severity of colds was not significant. Other studies have shown a similar pattern, that is, megadoses of vitamin C result in small but inconsistent decreases in the severity of symptoms. They do not affect the number of colds. Interestingly, younger children seem to benefit more than older children from vitamin C treatments.

Another study worth noting was conducted using school-age twins as subjects. One twin from each pair was given vitamin C, while the other was given a placebo, or inactive substance, with the same appearance and taste of the vitamin C. As twins living in the same household, they were exposed to all the same factors that could potentially influence a cold. Technically, this was a nearly ideal experiment. The results of this study were similar to those reported by other investigators: the children taking vitamin C had somewhat less severe colds, but the number was essentially the same. The effect was slightly greater among younger children.

Unfortunately, vitamin C has not been proven to cure or prevent the common cold. You might expect a mild reduction in cold symptoms, although doses as high as 1 g. do not seem to be necessary. Studies have been conducted in which 80–200 mg. per day were sufficient to produce this effect (a cup of orange juice contains 100–125 mg.). One cannot help but wonder whether the same minor benefits wouldn't be obtained by taking aspirin, a shot of whiskey, chicken soup, or any other home remedy.

It is possible that a small number of people are deficient in vitamin C or need unusually large amounts. These few people will be helped by taking extra vitamin C. But it does not make sense to consume large amounts of any drug for which a substantial benefit has not been demonstrated. We believe that a daily glass of orange juice or a multivitamin tablet taken during the cold season will do as much as any megadose of vitamin C and cost a lot less.

Cancer Treatment

Linus Pauling and Ewan Cameron reported in 1976 that cancer patients in Scotland who were treated with vitamin C lived an average of 210 days longer than 1,000 patients not given vitamin C, but there were serious technical problems with this study, including an inappropriate control population, that cast grave doubts about the conclusions drawn. In any scientific experiment, the best results are obtained when the two groups of subjects compared are as identical as possible in all ways except for the agent being tested, in this case vitamin C. Pauling and Cameron's patients were not compared against a control group of similar patients receiving treatments identical except for vitamin C. Instead, they were compared against the hospital records of 1000 past patients who the authors felt were comparable.

A 1979 study conducted at the Mayo Clinic could not confirm the findings of Pauling and Cameron; no benefit was detected from vitamin C therapy, although the cancer patients in this study had received prior drug treatment while those in the Pauling and Cameron study had not. Pauling and Cameron countered with the argument that drug therapy with anticancer drugs may have negated any effects of vitamin C therapy, since many anticancer drugs suppress the body's immune system, thus accounting for the inability of the Mayo Clinic group to reproduce their results. However, the usefulness of vitamin C for cancer is still in question.

Another recent study indicates that women with cervical disorders had a daily vitamin C intake of less than half the RDA. The researchers concluded that vitamin C supplements would protect these women from developing cervical cancer. While this conclusion is not warranted by the facts of the study, it does point out the importance of maintaining your daily RDA of vitamin C, especially since we know that vitamin C inhibits the conversion of nitrates, found in many foodstuffs as a preservative, to nitrosamines, a known cancer risk factor.

Reduction of Rectal Polyps

One report indicates that taking 3 g. a day of ascorbic acid for one year resulted in fewer polyps. Rectal polyps are outpouchings or bulges in tissues surrounding the rectum and should not be confused with hemorrhoids, which involve swollen and engorged blood vessels.

Considering the risk of colon cancer associated with rectal polyps, this finding may be very important, but more work needs to be done to define the usefulness of vitamin C in eliminating rectal polyps. Also, if vitamin C does reduce the number of polyps, the value of this therapy in reducing the incidence of rectal cancer would also need to be established. The preliminary results are very encouraging, and we would recommend that people with rectal polyps take megadoses of vitamin C. Remember, vitamin C is not a substitute for proper monitoring of your condition by a physician.

Alleviation of Mental Illness

Several researchers who investigated the role of ascorbic acid in the treatment of people who were anxious and depressed or who had a diagnosed mental illness reported that vitamin C offered relief from anxiety and tension. Others have pointed out that replacement of vitamin C in people suffering from mental illness—who are also vitamin deficient—will result in the improvement of symptoms. However, the data is still too scarce to support the outright use of megadoses of ascorbic acid in the treatment of mental illness.

Detoxifying Alcoholics and Drug Abusers

There are a small number of unverified reports attesting to the usefulness of enormous doses of ascorbic acid—in some cases given by injection—in drying out alcoholics and detoxifying people addicted to narcotics and tranquilizers. People treated with vitamin C are given massive doses (up to 85 g. a day; that's *85,000 mg.*!) and are supposed to experience fewer of the adverse effects normally associated with drug withdrawal: cramps, nausea, generalized discomfort. This application of vitamin C should be considered unproven, although future research may shed some light on a possible role for vitamin C in this regard.

Lowering of Cholesterol Level

The story of vitamin C and cholesterol is riddled with conflicting information. While there is agreement that ascorbic acid will lower blood cholesterol in vitamin-deficient patients, it does not necessarily follow that cholesterol levels in other people will be affected. In fact, more recent studies have shown that people with high blood cholesterol who are otherwise healthy are either not affected by vitamin C or may actually have their cholesterol levels raised by the vitamin! At this point, it seems we must look elsewhere for an effective cholesterol-lowering agent.

Healing of Bedsores

Pressure sores, or bedsores, are a source of severe discomfort and infection for people who are bedridden for prolonged periods of time. It has been reported that pressure sores healed faster when extra vitamin C was given, possibly because of the role played by C in collagen synthesis. A study conducted in England on twenty surgical patients showed an 84 percent reduction in the size of pressure sores after one month of treatment with doses of vitamin C ranging from 1 to 30 g. per day, compared with a 43 percent reduction in the group receiving no extra vitamin C. Again, these findings are encouraging but need confirmation.

Relief of Genital Herpes Infections

Since vitamin C has been shown to be of some benefit for herpes cold sores, one would think that vitamin C might also relieve painful genital herpes infections, caused by a related Herpes Simplex virus. Unfortunately, studies conducted at the University of Washington have failed to show any beneficial effect of the vitamin on genital herpes infections.

Prevention of Periodontal Disease

Of particular interest to many people is the question of periodontal (gum) disease that has been linked to even marginal deficiencies of vitamin C. Since even Cartier's original description of scurvy included a reference to bleeding gums and the loss of teeth, some researchers recommend that daily megadoses of vitamin C (1–3 g.) should be taken to prevent periodontal problems. We must reaffirm, however, that this conclusion is erroneous, unless the patient can be established as deficient in vitamin C.

Vitamin C has also been promoted for other uses for which its value has not been proven. We cannot recommend that you take this vitamin to treat arthritis, eye disease, fatigue, harden-ing of the arteries, heart disease, infertility, stomach bleeding, or Tay-Sachs disease. Vitamin C also will not improve academic or intellectual performance or lengthen your lifespan.

Availability

A stroll down the vitamin aisle of your local pharmacy, health food, or vitamin store will soon make you aware that ascorbic acid is available in just about every possible dosage form (tablet, capsule, liquid, syrup, natural, synthetic, crystals, chewable, timed-release, wafers) and strength (100 mg., 250 mg., 500 mg., 1,000 mg., 1,500 mg., 100 g., 500 g., 1,000 g.). We suggest you follow the guidelines laid out in Chapter 6 for product selection.

8

Fat-Soluble Vitamins

Vitamin A

Vitamin A is most familiar as a cure for night blindness. In fact, night blindness is a symptom of vitamin A deficiency which can be alleviated by taking in sufficient amounts of that vitamin.

Symptoms of night blindness were first recognized in ancient Egypt around 1500 B.C. Although the problem was not linked to a dietary deficiency of any kind, the symptoms were treated by placing roasted or fried liver over the eyes. Later, Hippocrates suggested eating beef liver—a rich source of vitamin A—as a cure for night blindness.

Today we know that vitamin A serves several other important functions in the human body and may have significant future medical benefits—particularly for cancer treatment.

This important vitamin is found in two forms. Vitamin A in animal tissues, called retinol, is "ready to go" and can be absorbed as is by the body. Vitamin A found in plants, called beta carotene, is considered a "provitamin" because it must be broken down in the body into retinol before it can act as a vitamin.

function

Vitamin A is essential to a variety of biochemical and physiological processes in the body. In many of these processes, the vitamin must undergo a minor chemical change to allow it to participate in that function.

Vitamin A, as retinal, is a part of the pigment called rhodopsin found in the retina of the eye. Rhodopsin is sensitive to small amounts of light and is essential for night vision because it allows us to discern objects in very low light. To function in this way, the retina of the eye must contain a large concentration of vitamin A.

Retinol participates in a number of chemical reactions that are a part of the manufacture of proteins essential to the maintenance of healthy skin. These same reactions are essential to the maintenance of function in other body cells that reproduce frequently. Vitamin A is necessary for the production of RNA, one of the architects of all body cells. As such, vitamin A is needed for normal bone growth, sperm cell production in men, and the growth of a fertilized egg into a healthy baby.

Vitamin A is thought to prevent some cancers, but the exact way that the vitamin exerts this effect is not known. Retinol may interfere with the activation of cancer-causing chemicals and their binding to DNA in the cell. Other possible mechanisms for an anticancer effect of vitamin A include interference with enzyme systems, an increase in the normal body system that repels cancer-causing substances, and a direct effect of the retinoid on the cancerous cell.

Daily Requirements

The strength of vitamin A can be expressed in terms of international units (IU), based on measure of biological activity, or as retinol equivalents (RE), which indicate the amount of retinol to which the substance can be converted in the body. One IU of vitamin A from carotene is equivalent to 1 IU of vitamin A as retinol. References and food or vitamin labels may express vitamin A activity either as IUs or REs. You can convert between systems simply by remembering that 1 RE of vitamin A equals 5 IU of vitamin A.

The adult RDA for vitamin A is 1,000 RE (5,000 IU) for men and 800 RE (4,000 IU) for women. Pregnant or breastfeeding women need an additional 200 and 400 RE (1,000 and 2,000 IU), respectively.

The RDA for infants and children is smaller than that for adults (400–700 RE or 2,000–3,500 IU). But when compared on a pound-for-pound basis, it is considerably larger because of the need for vitamin A in normal processes of growth and development.

Taking small amounts of vitamin E will increase the capacity of all body tissues, including the retina and liver, to store vitamin A. But, too much vitamin E will interfere with the absorption of vitamin A. For this reason, people who must take vitamin A to correct a deficiency state should accompany the A with modest amounts of vitamin E. Most comprehensive multivitamin formulas have enough vitamin E in them to satisfy this need for the vitamin.

However, it is essential to point out that there is no need for a person in good health to take a vitamin A supplement. A daily multivitamin with about 5,000 IU's of A is more than sufficient for the average person because the vitamin A received in the diet must also be taken into account.

Dietary Sources

If you remember that the retinols dissolve in fat and the carotenes are found in yellow plant pigments, it is easy to recall which foods are rich in vitamin A.

Some rich animal sources of vitamin A are liver, the storage depot for vitamin A in all animals, whole milk, cream, and butter. Additional good sources are listed in the accompanying table.

Four ounces of beef liver has more than a seven-day supply of vitamin A, and fish liver has even more. Cod liver oil was commonly used as a source of this vitamin and of vitamin D before purified vitamin A was available. Four ounces of cod liver oil has over 40,000 REs, or 200,000 IU, of vitamin A

Vitamin A Content of Selected Foods
Average adult RDA is 900 RE, or 4,500 IU.

Food	Approximate Content (IUs per 3 oz.)
Apricots	2,430
Asparagus	810
Butter	2,520
Broccoli	3,150
Cantaloupe	3,060
Carrots	9,000
Cheese	1,170
Cherries	900
Chicken	190
Cod	163
Corn	360
Crab	1,980
Cucumbers	175
Eggs	1,080
Endive	3,000
Green beans	540
Green peppers	380
Herring	135
Kumquats	540
Halibut	765
Lettuce (iceberg)	900
Lettuce (Romaine)	1,700
Liver (beef)	33,300
Lobster	828
Mackerel	400
Mango	1,620
Milk (low fat)*	155
Milk (whole)	200
Nectarine	1,440
Okra	470
Oranges	180
Oysters	280
Papaya	1,530
Peaches	1,170

Vitamin A Content of Selected Foods

Food	Approximate Content (IUs per 3 oz.)
Persimmons	2,430
Pimentos	2,070
Pistachios	205
Pumpkin	6,300
Soybeans	630
Spinach	7,200
Sprouts	495
Squash (summer)	360
Squash (winter)	3,600
Swordfish	1,890
Tomatoes	800
Walnuts	270
Watermelon	475
Whitefish	1,800

*Normally, Vitamin A is found in the milk fat, which is removed from skim milk. If the milk you buy is supplemented with vitamin A (not all are), it also has 200 IU in 3 oz.

activity; a single teaspoon will fulfill the adult RDA. High concentrations of carotene are found in dark green vegetables, where the green of chlorophyll usually covers the yellow-to-orange carotenoid color, and yellow-orange–colored vegetables such as carrots, pumpkin, and squash. Other rich sources are listed in the accompanying table.

Carotene is converted to retinol in the wall of the small intestine as it is being absorbed into the blood. The process of conversion continues only as long as more retinol is needed; once the need for retinol is satisfied, the conversion process stops.

Vitamin A is sensitive to oxygen; therefore prolonged heating in the presence of air will destroy the vitamin A activity of any food. To minimize this loss while cooking your food, put a small lid on the pan or pot used to boil such vegetables as squash or carrots and use a small pot with just enough water to cover the vegetables. Acid also destroys A, but most food sources of this vitamin are nonacidic, so this is not a practical problem.

Deficiencies

About 15 percent of Americans, mostly infants and children, are deficient in vitamin A intake. Fortunately, the average person has about a two-year supply of vitamin A in his or her liver, so you have to eat a vitamin A–deficient diet for many months before symptoms will develop.

Symptoms of Deficiency

Mild vitamin A deficiency may be easily overlooked. Dry, rough skin is common. Sometimes the skin can crack and may even become infected. Because of this, vitamin A has been called the anti-infective vitamin, a misnomer because it suggests that vitamin A supplements will protect against infection. In vitamin A deficiency, the infection develops because cracks and rough areas in the skin leave openings for microorganisms to enter.

The most recognizable sign of vitamin A deficiency is night blindness (difficulty seeing at night or in low light). This is followed by further damage to the cornea in the form of an ailment called xeropthalmia. If left untreated, severe vitamin A deficiency can lead to permanent blindness.

People who are vitamin A deficient have more respiratory infections because of changes in the mucous and cells that line the bronchioles and respiratory tract that increase susceptibility.

Hearing, taste, smell, and nerve damage and reduced sweat gland function may also occur.

Other possible effects of vitamin A deficiency include slow growth, thickening of bone, kidney stones that originate with changes in some of the cells which line the kidney tubules, diarrhea, infant malformations, and reduced production of steroid hormones in the body. Steroids are produced by the adrenal gland and are a part of your natural response to stress and your immune function. Failure to make these important hormones will leave your immune system in a less than ideal state.

It is possible to measure blood levels of vitamin A, but the results of this test are usually not useful for the following reason. Since we store vast amounts of vitamin A in the liver, it takes many months for the blood test to reflect a vitamin A deficiency. Thus, a blood test that shows normal vitamin A levels cannot indicate how much vitamin A is left in reserve and how severely we might need supplementation. A blood test that shows low vitamin A levels is a direct indication of severe vitamin deficiency that demands immediate attention.

Toxicity

Adults will develop symptoms of vitamin A toxicity after taking more than 50,000 IUs a day for long periods of time or after taking a single dose of 300,000 IUs or more.

Infants given 7,500–15,000 RE (37,500–75,000 IU) of vitamin A for thirty days have developed toxicity symptoms. In children, vitamin A toxicity has usually been caused by an overzealous parent combining large amounts of carotene-containing foods with excessive quantities of supplemental vitamin A. Infants and children who are given 6,000 RE (30,000 IU) of vitamin A a day and who eat a reasonable diet are likely to develop overdose symptoms after one or two months.

Interestingly, taking vitamin E appears to protect against vitamin A toxicity because it increases the capacity of body tissues to store vitamin A. But, too much vitamin E interferes with the absorption of A.

Vitamin A overdose is characterized by vomiting, fatigue, swelling due to fluid accumulation, hydrocephalus (water on the brain), and headache (caused by excess fluid in the skull, resulting in increased pressure on the brain). Vitamin A overdose has, in some cases, been misdiagnosed as a brain tumor.

Other symptoms of overdose are liver and lymph gland enlargement, difficulty sleeping, joint pains, constipation, and rough skin.

Since the body will convert as much carotene to retinol as it needs, it is possible to have excess unconverted carotene in the blood. A very high concentration of unconverted carotene in the blood is known as hypercarotenemia and can cause a yellow discoloration of the skin. This condition has been confused with jaundice, but the two are not related. The effects of an overdose of vitamin A will usually reverse themselves after you stop taking the vitamin.

Toxicity and Pregnant Women

Pregnant women taking excessive amounts of vitamin A risk birth defects because of the action of the vitamin on the developing fetus. Some of the possible defects are urinary tract malformations, water on the brain, and bone deformities. If you are pregnant, do not exceed your doctor's recommendations for daily supplements of vitamin A, or any other vitamin.

Interactions

In addition to its interaction with vitamin E, discussed above, vitamin A can also interact with corticosteroid-type drugs used for inflammation, oral contraceptives, calcium, zinc, and mineral oil. It can also interfere with certain blood tests. See Part IV, "Vitamin, Mineral and Drug Interactions," for details.

Therapeutic Uses

Vitamin A supplements may be given to counteract any of the standard symptoms of vitamin A deficiency reviewed earlier in the profile. However, such symptoms will not be alleviated by vitamin A unless they are, in fact, caused by vitamin deficiency.

In addition, compounds with vitamin A activity have greater potential than any other vitamin for future medical benefits, and pharmaceutical companies are spending millions of dollars on research into this vitamin.

Most successful to date is a vitamin A derivative called retinoic acid. Retinoic acid compounds were developed by researchers with the aim of increasing vitamin A activity and decreasing toxic effect. Only small amounts of retinoic acid are present in the body, and we don't store it, unlike retinol, which is present in large quantities and stored in the liver.

Retinoic acid is carried in the blood by a different protein (retinoic acid binding protein, or RAPB) than the one which binds retinol and carries it in the blood (retinol binding protein, or RBP). Many of the more promising derivatives of retinoic acid are not even carried by RABP; they are bound to albumin, the most common blood protein. Since retinoic acids are not stored in the body or carried by RBP, they are more specific in their effect and safer.

The following are some conditions for which vitamin A therapy seems hopeful. But remember, vitamin A in recommended doses is not strong enough to benefit these conditions, and if you take too much, it can be dangerous. Unfortunately, the more potent but less toxic vitamin A compounds and derivatives will not be commercially available for some time.

Cancer Treatment

Animals with vitamin A deficiency get cancer more often and their tumors spread more quickly than animals without this deficiency. There is some evidence that the same thing holds true for human beings; people who are deficient in vitamin A may be at increased risk of developing cancer and their cancer may spread more quickly.

In 1982, the National Research Council issued a report entitled *Diet, Nutrition and Cancer*. In that report, vitamin A deficiency was directly related to an increase in cancer of the lung, bladder, and larynx. However, it is not known whether the protective effect of vitamin A is caused by carotene, retinol, vitamin A, or some other component of green and yellow vegetables.

Surveys conducted in Norway revealed that smokers with diets deficient in vitamin A had twice as much lung cancer as smokers whose vitamin A intake was not deficient. At first, these patients were treated with high doses of vitamin A, but they suffered from side effects of this therapy before any effect on their cancer could be documented. Similar results have been reported from Japan, Singapore, and the United States. When researchers started experimenting with retinoic acid derivatives, they found these compounds to be stronger and less toxic for cancer treatment.

Many studies undertaken to observe the relationship between cancer and the consumption of vitamin A–containing foods, such as green and yellow vegetables, have shown that people who ate less of these foods were more likely to have cancer than would otherwise be expected. Also, cancer patients have been found to have low blood levels of carotene. However, this observation is not consistent in all studies, possibly because of the difficulty in obtaining matched groups of people and keeping adequate food intake records. Some find no significant relationship between vitamin A and cancer.

There is little chance for the development of a "magic bullet" that will cure all cancers. Nevertheless, retinoic acid compounds are promising drugs and will most likely be used together with other weapons against cancer.

Treatment of Acne

One of the symptoms of vitamin A deficiency is an acnelike condition. This observation led to the use of vitamin A capsules as an acne treatment in the 1950s and 1960s and led to the discovery that high doses of vitamin A are toxic. After a decade of using vitamin A capsules to treat acne, the consensus of opinion is that the treatment is only marginally effective.

In the 1970s, topical retinoic acid became popular as an acne treatment and is still used today. When applied to the skin, retinoic acid appears to reduce the plugging of sebaceous (oil-producing) glands. Plugged sebaceous glands can become infected and turn into pimples. Retinoic acid also mildly irritates the skin and causes peeling, which also helps to free plugged sebaceous glands.

Retinoic acid cream or lotion applied to the skin is not the ideal treatment. It can take months for the treatment to take effect and is irritating to the skin. In the search for more potent and less toxic retinoic acid derivatives, researchers have discovered several that can be taken by mouth without the usual adverse effects. The first vitamin A derivative to become available for prescription use was 13-cis-retinoic acid, or isotretinoin. Now available under the brand name of Accutane, it has been of some benefit to people who suffer from the most severe form of acne and who have not responded to other forms of treatment.

Treatment of Psoriasis

Several studies using chemical derivatives of retinol, known as retinoids, in the treatment of psoriasis have been reported, and the results, to date, appear promising.

Unsubstantiated Claims

Vitamin A has also been promoted for other uses for which its value has not been proven. We cannot recommend that you take this vitamin to treat alcoholism, allergies, angina pectoris, arteriosclerosis, arthritis, asthma, bad breath, broken bones, bronchitis, canker sores, cataracts, colitis, the common cold, constipation, cystitis, diabetes, diarrhea, double vision, ear infections, emphysema, epilepsy, eye strain, fever, flu, gout, hair problems, hay fever, headache, heartattack, heart failure, hemorrhoids, hemophilia, hepatitis, infertility, jaundice, kidney stones, learning disabilities, liver cirrhosis, meningitis, mononucleosis, muscular dystrophy, nail problems, osteomalacia, prostate trouble, psychoses, sinusitis, stroke, swollen glands, thyroid disease, tuberculosis, vaginitis, varicose veins, or worms.

Availability

Vitamin A toxicity is not a trivial illness. Because of this, the U.S. Food and Drug Administration limits the vitamin A products sold without a prescription to a maximum of 2,000 RE (10,000 IU) per dosage unit (tablet, capsule, teaspoon, etc.). Some vitamin A advocates have objected to this policy as being overprotective, but the potential for toxic effects makes this a necessary regulation to protect the general public.

Vitamin D

You can satisfy your vitamin D requirement simply by being out in the sun. That's why vitamin D is commonly called the sunshine vitamin.

Until discovery of vitamin D in 1924, many urban children suffered from rickets, a crippling bone disease resulting from insufficient calcium. Some thought that rickets was caused by a lack of sunshine and fresh air, while others felt a dietary factor was responsible for this problem. By 1920, it was shown that both notions were true. Either cod liver oil, which contains large amounts of both vitamins A and D, or exposure to sunlight will prevent or cure the disease.

The term *vitamin D* describes two substances with the ability to increase the absorption of calcium into the bloodstream from the intestine. The first substance, now called vitamin D_3, or cholecalciferol, is made in the body from cholesterol that has been exposed to the ultraviolet light rays of direct sunlight. Electric lights do not give off the kind of light needed to convert cholesterol to vitamin D_3—you must be exposed directly to the sun. Sitting behind a window on a sunny day is also insufficient because the glass absorbs ultraviolet rays.

The second form, called vitamin D_2, or ergocalciferol, is made in the laboratory by exposing ergosterol, a fatty substance found in plants, to ultraviolet light. Vitamin D_2 is the form used for food fortification. Both D_2 and D_3 are equally potent; your body can use either form.

function

Vitamin D is best described as a regulator of calcium metabolism in the body. In fact, vitamin D is so important to calcium function that many researchers consider it a hormone, not a vitamin.

The two most important ways that vitamin D functions to maintain normal calcium metabolism are the absorption of calcium through the intestines into the bloodstream and the mobilization of calcium from bone, where 95 percent of body calcium is stored. In addition, vitamin D exerts a direct effect on the kidneys to prevent the release of calcium and phosphates from the body via the urine. Although vitamin D has not been shown to influence the addition of calcium to bone directly, it does influence other body processes that depend on calcium, including nerve, muscle, and heart function and blood clotting.

Both the vitamin D that you convert in the skin after exposure to sunlight and that which you get from your diet must be converted to an active form called calcitriol, and both the liver and kidneys are involved in this process. Liver disease does not impede the conversion, but kidney failure is serious because less than optimal amounts of calcitriol are then produced, leading to calcium deficiency symptoms.

Daily Requirements

The strength of vitamin D is expressed in terms of international units (IU), based on measures of biological activity.

One hundred IUs of vitamin D per day is probably all that is needed to prevent deficiency symptoms, but 400 IUs is the value recommended as the RDA for most people. Few people need to take more than that, and people who live in the Sunbelt and expose themselves to the sun probably don't need any.

On the average, we make 6 IU of vitamin D every hour for every square inch of skin exposed to the sun. This varies because people whose skin color is darker make less vitamin D. People with a very dark skin color make about 4 IU per square inch per hour because less light is able to penetrate the skin to the layer where the conversion is carried out.

Dietary Sources

While sunshine provides sufficient amounts of vitamin D for people who live in warm and sunny climates, those who live in northern areas with fewer days of sunshine and extended periods of cloud cover and darkness have to depend on dietary sources for vitamin D.

Milk is one of our major dietary sources of vitamin D because it is fortified with irradiated ergosterol to provide vitamin D activity equivalent to 400 IU (or 10 mcg.) per quart. Fortified margarine is also very high in vitamin D. Additional food sources are listed in the accompanying table.

Vitamin D Content of Selected Foods
Average Adult RDA is 400 IU, or 10 mcg.

Food	Approximate Content (IU per 3 oz.)
Butter	36
Cheese	27
Cod liver oil	20,000
Eggs	45
Liver	45
Margarine (fortified)	270
Milk (fortified)	36
Milk (human)	6
Mushrooms	135
Salmon	360
Sardines	450
Shrimp	135
Sunflower seeds	83
Tunafish	225

Vitamin D is chemically stable and survives the usual modes of food processing.

Deficiencies

When a growing child is deficient in vitamin D, he or she develops rickets, a disease in which newly formed bone lacks calcium.

Vitamin D–deficient adults may develop osteomalacia, or adult rickets. Osteomalacia is most likely to occur during times of increased calcium need, such as pregnancy. It also occurs in some elderly people and people with kidney failure. Until recently, people with kidney failure had to take enormous amounts of vitamin D_2 to maintain normal calcium levels, and frequently even this was not enough. Now, the active form of vitamin D, calcitriol, which does not have to be converted in the body, is available on a prescription-only basis.

Symptoms of Deficiency

In rickets, defective bone is especially likely to form at sites of active growth. This results in bent, bowed legs, late tooth development, weak muscles, and listlessness.

In osteomalacia, there is a generalized loss of calcium from bones throughout the body, leaving large areas of porous, brittle bone without calcium to strengthen the matrix. Osteomalacia must be distinguished from osteoporosis, in which calcium is also lost from bones, but the losses are not general in nature— they are isolated in specific locations in the skeleton.

It is possible to measure vitamin D in the blood, but the procedure is used only for research purposes.

Toxicity

Vitamin D can be toxic if taken in large doses and should never be taken in daily doses larger than 400 IU per day, except when prescribed by your doctor to treat a specific condition. In adults, single doses of 150,000 IU or more are toxic, and daily doses of 2,000 IU or more taken on a regular basis can lead to abnormally high blood calcium levels. Now that vitamin D is more widely used as a treatment for osteoporosis, toxicity is more common among older women. Infants taking more than

400 IU per day on a regular basis may experience symptoms of toxicity.

Symptoms of toxicity are: weakness, tiredness, headache, nausea and vomiting, loss of appetite, constipation or diarrhea, excessive thirst and urination, protein in the urine, high blood pressure, high blood cholesterol, premature hardening of the arteries, mental retardation, and slower than normal growth. In addition, calcium may become deposited in vital tissues, leading to serious consequences such as liver damage and kidney failure.

Interactions

Vitamin D can interact with phenytoin taken for seizures, barbiturates, and minerals and can interfere with certain blood tests. See Part IV, "Vitamin, Mineral, and Drug Interactions."

Therapeutic Uses

Vitamin D supplements may be given to counteract the symptoms of vitamin D deficiency reviewed earlier in this profile. However, such symptoms will not be alleviated by vitamin D unless they are, in fact, caused by vitamin deficiency.

In addition to the prevention and treatment of the deficiency diseases, rickets and osteomalacia, vitamin D may also be used to treat people whose parathyroid gland is not properly functioning. The parathyroid is involved in the regulation of calcium use by the body: when the blood level of calcium is low, the parathyroids release a hormone that stimulates the kidneys to convert vitamin D to its active form, calcitriol, which in turn stimulates the absorption of more calcium through the intestines and the removal of some calcium from bones, until the level is acceptable. An improperly functioning parathyroid will not stimulate the conversion of vitamin D to calcitriol.

Plain vitamin D may be used to treat this condition, but people often do not respond to even larger doses of the vitamin. Other vitamin D derivatives, dihydrotachysterol (DHT) or calcitrol (Rocaltrol), are more effective in drawing calcium out of bone than the plain vitamin and are used as the treatment for people who do not respond to plain vitamin D.

Conditions associated with low blood levels of phosphate, such as Fanconi syndrome, are treated with vitamin D as well.

Vitamin D draws phosphate out of bone along with some calcium and can help to restore normal phosphate levels.

Unsubstantiated Claims

Vitamin D has also been promoted for other uses for which its value has not been proven. We cannot recommend that you take this vitamin to treat: acne, aging symptoms, alcoholism, allergies, arthritis, backache, bed sores, blood cholesterol, broken bones, bronchitis, burns, cancer, canker sores, carbuncles, cataracts, the common cold, constipation, cystic fibrosis, cystitis, diabetes, eczema, emphysema, epilepsy, eye strain, fatigue, fever, gallstones, glaucoma, herpes simplex, herpes zoster, jaundice, leg cramps, liver cirrhosis, meningitis, osteoporosis, psoriasis, pyorrhea, rheumatic fever, sciatica, sleeplessness, stress, tuberculosis, vaginitis, or worms.

Availability

Vitamin D, at a dose of 400 IU, is an ingredient of virtually every multivitamin formula. Products containing more than 400 IU of vitamin D per dosage unit are available only on prescription.

Vitamin E

Despite intense research, the true function of vitamin E is still a mystery. While most scientists agree that vitamin E plays a role in biochemical processes that protect us from some of the effects of oxygen, there is disagreement on whether its action is direct or indirect.

A host of medical uses for vitamin E have been advanced, including treatment for infertility. This is based on discoveries in the 1920s that a specific dietary component (vitamin E) was necessary for female rats to sustain a normal pregnancy; vitamin E–deficient rats would ovulate and conceive, but their pregnancies were never completed. Vitamin E–deficient male rats were found to have lesions on their testicles. However, rats and humans are not the same, and there is no basis for E's popularity as the "antisterility" vitamin.

Many other claims reviewed in this profile are based on incomplete evidence, unsubstantiated testimonials, and equally faulty reasoning. It is possible that some of the proposed applications for vitamin E may prove to be of benefit at some time in the future, but they cannot be considered realistic at this time.

In human nutrition, the important form of vitamin E is alpha tocopherol, and the natural form of this substance is alpha tocopherol. Synthetic alpha tocopherol contains half of the natural form and half of another form, l-alpha tocopherol, plus an acetate group to stabilize the vitamin E. Dl-alpha tocopherol acetate is therefore the name for the fifty-fifty mixture.

Function

Oxygen is life-giving, but it can also be harmful. Vitamin E helps to prevent it from causing serious damage to the body.

One of the most potentially damaging reactions in which oxygen is involved is with unsaturated fatty acids. This combination can form substances called organic peroxides, which are toxic to body cells. In effect, the oxygen converts fluidlike unsaturated fatty acids to inactive solids that can cause cellular death. One of nature's protective mechanisms against this is vitamin E, which works to neutralize this effect.

There is a lot of research to support this role for vitamin E. For instance, people who consume more polyunsaturated fat in their diet require more vitamin E to prevent a deficiency state. A relative absence of vitamin E in the diet may lead to the deposition of solidified fatty acids in body tissues. Interestingly, these solids are similar to the pigments in liver spots that are commonly associated with the aging process in both animals and people. That is not to say that vitamin E will prevent aging (it will not), but it is possible that vitamin E deficiency will speed the aging of essential tissues.

Daily Requirements

The strength of vitamin E was originally expressed in terms of international units (IU) based on measures of biological activity. Dl-alpha tocopherol acetate was assigned a potency of 1 IU per mg. and Dl-alpha tocopherol without the acetate a potency of 1.1 IU per mg. The natural form of the vitamin, d-alpha tocopherol, was equaled to 1.5 IU per mg. In 1980, the RDA for vitamin E was changed from IU to alpha tocopherol equivalents (TE). One TE is equivalent to 1.5 IU.

Based on early studies, an RDA of 30 IU per day was set in 1968. In 1974, the National Research Council reduced the RDA to 15 IU, which is 10 TE. This was done on the basis of dietary surveys which revealed that most diets contained between 10 and 15 IU per day. Since there were no obvious signs of vitamin E deficiency in America, it was assumed that the previous recommendation was too high.

This decision was extremely controversial. On one hand, there was no evidence that 15 IU per day will not satisfy human needs for the vitamin. On the other hand, animal studies indicate that, as we eat more unsaturated fats, our need for E increases. Critics of the National Research Council action also note that we are eating more and more refined foods in which much of the vitamin E has been destroyed by processing techniques.

The controversy is still unresolved. While it would be hard to eat a diet that would provide more than 30 IU of vitamin E, it seems prudent to increase our consumption of whole grain and unprocessed foods to increase vitamin E intake.

Practically speaking, the body doesn't care whether vitamin E is obtained from natural or synthetic sources, as long as the equivalent IUs are provided. All available evidence indicates that 1 IU of synthetic vitamin E is just as effective as 1 IU of the natural form of the vitamin. Synthetic E may even have an advantage because of the acetate attached to it, which keeps the molecule stable for long periods of time. Once consumed, the body easily removes the acetate and feeds it into our metabolic machinery. Other forms of vitamin E found in nature have less than 10 percent of the activity of d-alpha tocopherol and are, therefore, of little interest.

Dietary Sources

Tocopherols are made by plants, probably as protection against oxidation of their vital fatty acids. Animals pick up their tocopherols from plant sources and use them as protection from the adverse effects of oxygen. Unlike vitamins A and D, which are stored only in body fat and the liver, vitamin E is found in all body tissues.

Some of our vitamin E comes from animal sources, but over 60 percent of the dietary vitamin E consumed in the United States comes from plants, especially from corn or cottonseed oil (in margarine), green vegetables, and wheat germ. Other good sources are listed in the accompanying table.

Vitamin E Content of Selected Foods
Average Adult RDA is 10 TE, or 15 IU.

Food	Approximate Content (IU per 3 oz.)
Almonds	13.5
Almond oil	5.8
Apricot oil	19.0
Brazil nuts	5.9
Cabbage	6.4
Cashew nuts	4.6
Corn oil	19.0
Cottonseed oil	40.0
Hazelnuts	19.0
Margarine	16.2
Peanuts	6.3
Peanut oil	14.4
Safflower nuts	31.5
Sunflower seeds	28.0
Walnuts	20.0
Wheat germ	144.0
Whole wheat flour	27.0

Vitamin E is the only vitamin destroyed by freezing (it is oxidized during the processing and storage). It also does not stand up under extreme heat.

Deficiencies

One perplexing feature of vitamin E is that while a vitamin E–deficient diet is life threatening to animals, man is not as severely affected. Vitamin E–deficient animals develop symptoms such as sterility, liver damage, muscular dystrophy, heart degeneration, and anemia, but no such deficiency symptoms exist for man.

A true human vitamin E deficiency state was not discovered until the 1960s, when a group of premature infants was accidentally given formula deficient in this vitamin. The infants became anemic and developed edema (swelling) that responded to vitamin E treatments. In Illinois, a group of volunteers was given a diet containing low levels of vitamin E. These studies showed that red blood cells from normal patients survived from 8 to 10 percent longer than those who were vitamin E deficient. There were no other obvious deficiency signs in the volunteers. The findings of this study, which originally set out to determine how much vitamin E would be needed to return the volunteers' red blood cells to normal, led to the 1968 recommendation by the Food and Nutrition Board to set the RDA at 30 IUs of vitamin E.

We assume that consuming a diet deficient in vitamin E for prolonged periods of time would have adverse consequences and would likely affect the stability of vital membranes, such as those of red blood cells. However, it is likely that humans have a backup system not available to animals to take the place of vitamin E.

Toxicity

There have been no significant adverse effects associated with taking vitamin E but it is involved in several important drug interactions. One of the best evaluations of vitamin E toxicity was conducted at the National Institutes of Health and reported in 1975. Twenty-eight institute employees voluntarily took 100–800 IU a day for an average of three years. A battery of tests designed to uncover possible toxic effects was performed on each volunteer and none were found. There are a few reports in medical literature describing possible stomach upset, diarrhea, dizziness, and increased blood clotting time with vitamin E, but most will agree that vitamin E is nontoxic.

One final note of caution: The long-term effects of taking megadoses of vitamin E in excess of those tested are not known.

Interactions

Small amounts of Vitamin E facilitates the absorption, tissue storage, and utilization of vitamin A. People who must take vitamin A to correct a deficiency should also take vitamin E. Large doses of vitamin E will interfere with the absorption of vitamin A into body tissues.

Vitamin E can also interact with oral anticoagulant drugs and iron. See Part IV, "Vitamin, Mineral, and Drug Interactions."

Therapeutic Uses

In spite of the fact that vitamin E has an unusually large number of unfounded claims to fame, it would be shortsighted to suggest that it has no therapeutic merit at all. Following is a discussion of some areas where vitamin E shows promise of being beneficial.

Protection of the Body from the Effects of Oxygen

There are several conditions where vitamin E may be useful in this role. In each case, more study is needed, but preliminary evidence suggests that vitamin E may be helpful for:

• Environmental hazards such as lead poisoning
• The cardiac toxicities of the anticancer drugs daunomycin and adriamycin
• Hemolytic anemia associated with a hereditary deficiency of the enzyme known as G6-PD
• Hereditary deficiency of the enzyme glutathione synthetase, which can lead to excess oxygen and consequent damaging of body tissues.
• Prevention of lung damage in infants given oxygen in the hospital.

Treatment of Cystic Breast Disease

Noncancerous breast lumps affect millions of American women. If vitamin E is proven beneficial in the treatment of cystic breast disease, it will be the first legitimate large-scale medical use for the vitamin. The lumps of cystic breast disease are sometimes painful and almost always worrisome because of the fear of malignancy. Indeed, some kinds of breast cysts sharply increase the risk for developing breast cancer. Clearly, we need a safe and effective treatment for this malady.

It is probably too soon to know just how useful vitamin E will be, but the results of a study conducted by one group of investigators at the Johns Hopkins School of Medicine in Baltimore are encouraging. In the 1980 study, women with a history of cystic breast disease were found to experience fewer attacks with vitamin E treatment and had fewer cysts. The majority of women in the study responded to treatment, and some achieved complete disappearance of the lumps and relief from pain. The dose of vitamin E used in the study was 600 IU per day taken for eight weeks. It is not known whether this is the optimal dose or whether more or less vitamin E is best for cystic breast disease.

Relief of Intermittent Severe Leg Muscle Pains (Intermittent Claudication)

Intermittent claudication is characterized by attacks of lameness and pain brought on by walking. The pain comes from narrowed arteries in the leg which are unable to provide sufficient amounts of oxygen to the calf and buttock muscles. The traditional treatments for this condition are anticoagulant medicines (blood thinners) and drugs that dilate (widen) the blood vessels and make it easier for blood to flow through them to the muscles. Tests to evaluate vitamin E measured the exercise tolerance of patients receiving the vitamin compared with people who received traditional treatment and others receiving no treatment at all. One study actually measured blood flow to the legs.

By all criteria, vitamin E was shown to be of some benefit after six months of continuous use. Vitamin E in megadoses (more than 1,000 IU per day) deserves more study as a treatment for circulation diseases in the arms and legs, especially for those who do not respond to other, more traditional treatments.

Relief of Nighttime Leg Cramps

The evidence suggests that vitamin E might offer some benefit to those who suffer from this annoying affliction, but long-term studies on the effectiveness of vitamin E for this problem have not been done. In one of the few published reports of the effect of vitamin E on nighttime leg cramps, 400 IU, taken before bed, was effective in reducing the frequency and severity of attacks.

Healing of Wounds

Although this use of vitamin E has not been scientifically tested, many people claim to have experienced great benefit from applying vitamin E creams or the oil from vitamin E capsules directly to wounds and scars. Vitamin E cream is a cosmetically elegant, more expensive way of applying the vitamin to your skin than simply using the oil from a vitamin E capsule, which can be removed by simply puncturing the capsule with a pin and squeezing it out. Either form of the vitamin should be applied to the wound or scar two or three times a day.

Although the mechanism by which vitamin E is supposed to hasten the healing process is not known, the vitamin would presumably work best when applied to a wound that has closed and is starting to heal. There are few adverse effects to this remedy, as long as you don't rub the cream or oil directly into an open wound. If you have a stubborn wound that is not healing as fast as you would like, this controversial treatment may be worth a try. But you should remember that a sore which doesn't heal is a warning sign of cancer, so check with your physician if you have any doubts.

Unsubstantiated Claims

Proponents of vitamin E treatments have used animal studies demonstrating that a vitamin E deficiency resulted in sterility as a basis for the claim that vitamin E has aphrodisiac qualities and will improve reproductive function in people. Similarly, other symptoms of vitamin E deficiency in animals have been used to suggest additional uses for vitamin E in humans: a treatment for muscular dystrophy, heart degeneration, anemia, and so on. The fault with this reasoning is that vitamin E deficiency in humans does not cause any of these problems. It is wrong to suggest that because vitamin E–deficient rabbits develop muscular dystrophy, vitamin E will be an effective treatment for muscular dystrophy in humans.

There is no scientific evidence to support the claims discussed below. If vitamin E were the cure-all some proponents claim, it probably would have been discovered long before this!

Treatment of Heart Diseases

With little or no evidence to go on, megavitamin advocates have supported vitamin E as being beneficial, even lifesaving in the treatment of heart diseases. Careful studies conducted over the past twenty years have failed to support this enthusiasm.

The easiest heart disease with which to test vitamin E effectiveness is angina, or angina pectoris, which comes from the narrowing of arteries that supply blood to the heart muscle. As the flow of blood through these arteries becomes restricted, less food and oxygen are delivered and severe chest pains develop. Drug effectiveness is measured by the length of time patients can exercise before the pain becomes oppressive. Also, the number of nitroglycerin tablets required to relieve the anginal pain can be monitored. If a drug or treatment allows the patient to use fewer nitroglycerin, it is judged successful in preventing and/or treating angina. Studies using these techniques have shown vitamin E to be of no substantial benefit for this condition. A recent, well-designed study using megadoses of vitamin E has confirmed this conclusion.

Improvement of Sexual Function

Sorry folks, despite its reputation, vitamin E will not do anything for your sexual prowess. A Canadian evaluation could not demonstrate any effect of vitamin E on the sexual activities of couples when compared with a group receiving an inactive substance.

Improvement of Athletic Performance

Many athletes take extra vitamin E in the hope that it will improve their performance. Based on the vitamin's antioxygen properties, the premise is that vitamin E will prevent oxygen from reacting with vital body tissues. This will leave more oxygen to make energy, increasing athletic endurance and/or performance. Careful studies on student athletes in England and on members of a college swimming team in Louisiana have shown that vitamin E does not help.

Removal of Scars

There are people who claim that vitamin E treatments will remove scars. To date, no scientific studies have been undertaken to test this theory, and until such data is available, we suggest that you let your body exert its remarkable biochemistry to heal cuts, scratches, and other abrasions.

Vitamin E has also been promoted for other uses for which its value has not been proven. We cannot recommend that you take this vitamin to treat: acne, allergies, anemia, arteriosclerosis, arthritis, athlete's foot, backache, baldness, bedsores, boils, bronchitis, bursitis, cancer, cataracts, colitis, the common cold, constipation, cystic fibrosis, cystitis, dandruff, diabetes, fluid retention, emphysema, epilepsy, eye strain, fatigue, gallstones, gout, hay fever, headache, heart failure, impetigo, hemorrhoids, high blood pressure, infertility, impotence, kidney stones, loss of vision, measles, Meniere's disease, mental illness, menstrual cramps, multiple sclerosis, muscular dystrophy, nephritis, night blindness, obesity, osteoporosis, Parkinson's disease, phlebitis, premenstrual syndrome, prostatitis, sciatica, sinusitis, stroke, sunburn, thyroid disease, ulcers, vaginitis, or warts.

Vitamin E will also not increase virility or breast size, help avoid miscarriage, prevent skin wrinkles, or delay or reverse aging.

Availability

Capsules and tablets of vitamin E are available without a prescription in strengths ranging from 30 to 1,000 IU. Vitamin E ointments, lotions, and creams are also available without a prescription. The usual concentration of vitamin E in these products is 30 IU per gram or 850 IU per ounce.

Vitamin K

You cannot form a blood clot unless vitamin K is present. This was discovered by a Danish doctor experimenting with the diet of chickens who bled spontaneously. He named this vitamin after the Danish word *koagulation*.

The term *vitamin K* refers to a series of compounds with similar chemical structures. The most important and useful vitamin K compound found in plants is called phytonadione, or vitamin K_1. Bacteria in our intestinal tract make a group of compounds known as menaquinones, or vitamin K_2. Menaquinones provide much of our daily vitamin K requirement. Vitamin K_3, called menadione, can be chemically produced in the laboratory. All of the vitamin K's—K_1, K_2, and K_3—dissolve in body fat, and some people who have trouble absorbing dietary fat into their bodies must take vitamin K supplements. To help these people, injectable and water-soluble forms of vitamin K have been developed.

Function

Blood clotting is a complex process involving at least eleven factors, each of which is necessary for a clot to form. Vitamin K is needed to make the active form of clotting factors II, VII, IX, and X.

Some research suggests that vitamin K also plays a role in the formation of bones during the growth and development of an unborn baby.

Daily Requirements

There are no official standards for daily vitamin K intake; however, our need for this important vitamin has been estimated by the Food and Nutrition Board of the National Academy of Sciences at about 12 mcg. per day for infants up to six months and 10–20 mcg. per day from six months to one year. Children's requirements vary with age and can be found in Table 1. The adult requirement is estimated at 70–150 mcg. per day.

At least half of our daily requirement of vitamin K is provided by bacteria normally found in our intestines, and the rest is provided via dietary means. An average diet provides at least ten times the amount thought to be needed for efficient blood clotting. The only exception to this rule is the newborn infant.

Infants are born with no vitamin K making bacteria in their

intestines, and all newborns are therefore given 0.5–1 g. (500–1,000 mcg.) of vitamin K immediately after birth to prevent a gradual decline in clotting factors over the days following birth and to prevent possible bleeding. The dose may have to be repeated if the mother had been taking anticoagulant or anticonvulsant medicines or if the infant develops a bleeding tendency. The clotting factors begin to rise to normal levels after about a week, when the necessary bacteria take up residence in the intestine..

Dietary Sources

Vitamin K is found in a variety of plants and other food sources. Brussels sprouts, spinach, cabbage, cauliflower, soy-

Vitamin K Content of Selected Foods
Estimated safe and adequate intake for adults is 70–150 mcg. per day.

Food	Approximate Content (mcg. per 3 oz.)
Alfalfa	470
Asparagus	50
Bran	62
Broccoli	180
Brussels sprouts	1,350
Cabbage	225
Camembert cheese	14,500
Cauliflower	250
Cheddar cheese	20,000
Coffee beans	35
Green tea	640
Lettuce	116
Liver, beef	81
Oats	440
Peas	40
Potatoes	72
Soybeans	270
Spinach	300
Turnip greens	585
Watercress	54

beans, Cheddar, and Camembert cheeses are particularly rich sources. Additional good sources are listed in the accompanying table.

Vitamin K is not harmed by normal storage and cooking processes.

Deficiencies

During their first five months of life, infants are vulnerable to a bleeding tendency if they were not given vitamin K at birth, and diarrhea or antibiotics that kill bacteria in the intestine can make things worse for infants with an already inadequate intake of vitamin K. Breastfed infants are more likely to develop a bleeding tendency than bottle-fed babies because breast milk contains little vitamin K and the intestinal bacteria of infants who are exclusively breastfed apparently lack the ability to make vitamin K. Formulas with cow's milk do contain sufficient amounts of vitamin K.

Vitamin K deficiency is rare in adults and usually occurs only in people who do not have enough bile to absorb this fat-soluble vitamin and must receive supplemental K by injection.

Symptoms of Deficiency
People with a vitamin K deficiency may experience nose bleeds, blood in the urine, stomach bleeding, and many small black and blue marks on the skin. It is not uncommon for a person with vitamin K deficiency to vomit blood.

Toxicity

Despite the fact that vitamin K is a fat-soluble vitamin, it is not stored in the body in large quantities, and that which is stored in body tissues is slowly destroyed.

Vitamin K preparations can, however, have some side effects. Newborns given vitamin K may develop a condition called hyperbilirubinemia, or excess bilirubin in the blood, leading to a form of jaundice that can cause brain damage or even death. Vitamin K_1 should be used for infants because it is the least likely to cause side effects.

Allergic reactions in the form of itching and rash, upset

stomach, nausea, and vomiting have also been reported in people taking vitamin K supplements.

Interactions

Vitamin K can interact with oral anticoagulant drugs to decrease their effect. Therefore, if you are taking anticoagulant drugs, you should avoid foods high in vitamin K.

Therapeutic Uses

Because of its interaction with anticoagulant drugs, vitamin K is sometimes given as an antidote to these drugs. It is also used therapeutically in cases of prolonged intravenous feeding and in situations where antibiotics are administered to kill all microorganisms in the intestines.

Unsubstantiated Claims

Vitamin K has also been promoted for other uses for which its value has not been proven. We cannot recommend that you take this vitamin to treat: alcoholism, cancer, cirrhosis, cystic fibrosis, gallstones, hepatitis, jaundice, or ulcers. It will also not prevent aging.

Availability

All vitamin K products, except those that contain 100 mcg. per tablet, are available on a prescription-only basis because of the potential toxic reactions and the fact that, between the bacteria in our intestines and food sources of the vitamin, it is unusual to be deficient in this vitamin.

Do not take any form of vitamin K unless prescribed by a doctor.

9

Pseudovitamins

Choline

Choline cannot be considered a vitamin because there are no deficiency symptoms in man. It is, however, a nutrient.

Choline and lecithin, another nutrient, are used interchangeably for the same therapeutic functions. Lecithin is composed of choline, inositol, which is another pseudovitamin, and fatty acids, but it is primarily used as a source of choline.

Function

There are two important functions in which choline has a role. First, choline is a lipotropic agent, which means that it removes excess fat from the liver.

Second, choline participates in the body process that makes acetylcholine. Acetylcholine is one of the primary neurohormones in the body and controls many body functions. As a neurohormone, acetylcholine stimulates sensitive nerve endings to transmit an impulse. If sufficient amounts of acetylcholine were not present, those nerve endings could not function.

Daily Requirements

No daily requirements for choline have been established. The average American gets 400–900 mg. a day from dietary sources. Infant formulas are fortified with choline at 7 mg. for every 100 calories, the same concentration found in mother's milk.

Choline Content of Selected Foods

Food	Approximate Content (mg. per 3 oz.)
Asparagus	111
Brewer's yeast*	204
Cabbage	213
Caviar	459
Chickpeas	663
Eggs	425
Egg yolk	1,445
Green beans	289
Lamb	94
Lentils	604
Calf's liver	468
Potatoes	94
Rice	553
Soybeans	289
Soy lecithin	2,465
Spinach	204
Split peas	595
Sprouts	179
Sunflower seeds	187
Trout	74
Veal	85

*Equivalent to 18 teaspoons.

Dietary Sources

Rich dietary sources of choline include egg yolks, peas, beans, cabbage, spinach, and a variety of seeds. Additional good sources are listed in the accompanying table.

Deficiencies

Choline deficiency is of no concern because the liver can make choline from carbohydrate (sugar) molecules and because our diet is rich in choline and choline-containing substances, such as lecithin. There are no deficiency symptoms in man, although some animal species can suffer from lack of choline.

Since choline is found in every cell in the body, there is no test for choline deficiency.

Toxicity

The lethal dose of choline is estimated to be somewhere in the range of 200 to 400 g. (roughly 0.5–0.9 lb.). Single doses of up to 10 g. (10,000 mg.) have not produced any harmful effects.

Therapeutic Uses

Recently, choline has been promoted as a treatment for Alzheimer's disease, a disorder known to be related to a chemical imbalance in the brain. Researchers have established that people with Alzheimer's disease are deficient in acetylcholine. The theory in using choline is that by supplying huge amounts of that chemical, the body will make more acetylcholine and the disease will be reversed or prevented. Although this approach has been disappointing, a few people have shown minor improvement with choline therapy.

Unsubstantiated Claims

Treatment of Liver Damage

Choline has enjoyed some popularity as a treatment for liver damage caused by alcoholism. The thinking here is based on the early observations that lecithin, the major dietary source of choline, reversed liver damage in dogs. Alcoholism usually causes liver damage identified by the deposition of large amounts of fat, the same kind of damage that was reversed by lecithin as a source of choline in the dogs. But studies to prove that choline is effective for this purpose in man have not been able to show a consistently positive effect.

Lowering of Cholesterol Level

Choline in the form of lecithin has also been used to prevent the formation of cholesterol-containing atherosclerotic plaques in the arteries. These plaques result in hardening of the arteries, a term that describes the loss of flexibility and elasticity in arteries onto which the plaques have been lodged. Once that happens, heart pains (angina) or even a heart attack may follow.

So far, there is not enough information to support the claim that choline will reverse or prevent either the process of plaque formation or the deposition of those plaques onto artery walls. A more reasonable approach to preventing hardening of the arteries is to avoid eating large amounts of saturated fats such as lard, butter, and animal fat and to replace them with the more mobile polyunsaturated fats found in plant oils. The use of polyunsaturated fats has been established as a way to retard hardening of the arteries.

Choline has also been promoted for other uses for which its value has not been proven. We cannot recommend that you take choline to treat: constipation, dizziness, ear noises, eczema, glaucoma and other eye disorders, hair problems, headaches, hypertension, insomnia, kidney disease, low blood sugar, muscular dystrophy, multiple sclerosis, or strokes.

Availability

Choline tablets (310 mg. each) can be bought in vitamin centers. Choline can also be found as an ingredient in some "lipotropic" multivitamin formulas (Liptriad, Lipoflavinoid) along with inositol and other nutrients.

Inositol

Inositol should not be considered a vitamin because there is no evidence pointing to a definite human need for this nutrient. Deficiency symptoms develop only in some animals, not in man. Chemically, inositol is a derivative of glucose (sugar).

Function

Inositol seems to play a role similar to choline in the movement of fats out of the liver. It is also incorporated into the structure of cell membranes in the form of phosphatidylinositol.

Daily Requirements

No requirement for inositol has been established in humans.

Dietary Sources

Inositol can be found in a wide variety of foods, including beans, chickpeas, rice, lentils, veal, liver, sunflower seeds, and wheat germ. Additional good sources are listed in the accompanying table.

The average American gets about 1 g. (1,000 mg.) of inositol from dietary sources.

Deficiencies

There are no deficiency symptoms associated with lack of dietary inositol, probably because we can make this nutrient from glucose in the liver. Animals that were made inositol deficient through dietary restriction lost their body hair and developed fat deposits in their livers.

There are no direct tests for inositol deficiency.

Toxicity

Inositol is considered nontoxic, even in gram doses.

Inositol Content of Selected Foods

Food	Approximate Content (mg. per 3 oz.)
Beans	204
Chickpeas	646
Cantaloupe	102
Cabbage	81
Cauliflower	81
Cheeses	19
Fruits	68
Grapefruit	128
Lentils	349
Calf's Liver	289
Milk (cow's)	43
Milk (mother's)	78
Oats	272
Oranges	179
Peanuts	153
Peas	136
Pork	349
Potatoes	25
Rice	595
Strawberries	102
Sunflower seeds	128
Veal	289
Wheat germ	587
Yams	56

Therapeutic Uses

No therapeutic uses are known.

Unsubstantiated Claims

Inositol has been used to treat diseases in which fat metabolism may be deranged or in which it is desirable to mobilize fat deposits. Several studies have reported minimal successes with supplementary inositol, but the data are not sufficient to support the statement that inositol can actually help improve any of these conditions. Some of the ailments that can fall into this category are arteriosclerosis, high blood cholesterol, stroke, heart disease, cirrhosis, and dizziness.

Inositol has also been promoted for other uses for which its value has not been proven. We cannot recommend that you take inositol to treat: asthma, baldness, constipation, glaucoma, obesity, or stomach upset.

Availability

Capsules of inositol may be purchased in vitamin and health food outlets in strengths of 325 and 650 mg. Inositol is also included in some ''lipotropic'' multivitamin formulas (Lipotriad, Lipoflavinoid) with choline and other nutrients.

Para Aminobenzoic Acid (PABA)

PABA should be considered a pseudovitamin because it has no role in human nutrition. It is, in fact, a chemical that bacteria use as part of the process whereby they manufacture folic acid. Folic acid is then used by bacteria for cell replication, so PABA could, in a sense, be considered a vitamin for bacteria.

In 1938, Dr. G. Domagk was awarded the Nobel prize in medicine for his discovery of the mechanism of action of a PABA derivative called Prontosil. He found that this drug interfered with the ability of bacterial cells to utilize PABA and thus acted as an antibacterial agent. Subsequently over five thousand sulfa drugs—as this antibacterial group has come to be known—were synthesized and served as the basis for the first antibacterial age.

Function

PABA serves no function in humans, and there are therefore no daily requirements.

Dietary Sources

Few foods have been tested for their PABA content. Two that have are: liver (0.52 mg./3 oz.) and sunflower seeds (53 mg./3 oz.).

Deficiency

There are no symptoms associated with PABA deficiency.

Toxicity

Large oral doses of PABA supplements can cause nausea and vomiting.

Therapeutic Uses

The only substantiated therapeutic use of PABA is as a sunscreen. PABA is the best available sunscreen and has been included in almost every suntan product. When applied to the skin in sufficient concentrations, PABA can actually block out almost all of the sun's burning rays.

The reason for PABA's effectiveness in this role is not known.

Unsubstantiated Claims

PABA has been promoted for other uses for which its value has not been proven. We cannot recommend that you take PABA to treat: anemia, baldness, constipation, gray hair, headaches, or skin disorders.

Availability

Incredibly, PABA tablets can be purchased in vitamin and health food stores in strengths of 30 mg., 100 mg., 250 mg., and 500 mg.

B₁₅ (Pangamic Acid)

So far, research has not proven this chemical to be useful for anything. Certainly, it does not meet the criteria established for vitamins: it has no known role in human nutrition, and people do not develop deficiency symptoms if deprived of pangamic acid.

Pangamic acid was discovered in apricot kernels along with laetrile by Russian biochemists. Dr. Ernest Krebs, Jr., promotes B₁₅ as an agent for speeding up metabolism and hence useful for athletes, the obese, and people with anemia. It has been used widely in the Soviet Union but has gained relatively little popularity in the United States.

True pangamic acid is a combination of gluconic acid and dimethylglycine. Commercial forms of pangamic acid may also contain sodium gluconate, glycine, dichloroacetate, diisopropylamine, or diisopropyl ammonium chloride.

Function

Advocates of pangamic acid claim that this substance enhances the delivery to and use of oxygen by body tissues, especially heart and other muscle, where it is said to promote the metabolism of protein. They also claim that pangamic acid regulates fat and sugar metabolism.

Daily Requirements

No daily requirement has been established for pangamic acid.

Dietary Sources

Pangamic acid can be found in apricot pits, wheat germ, and grains. Only a few other foods have been analyzed for their pangamic acid content; some of these are barley (10 mg./3 oz.), corn (128 mg./3 oz.), rice bran (170 mg./3 oz.), oats (94 mg./3 oz.), and wheat germ (60 mg./3 oz.).

Deficiencies

There are no known symptoms of pangamic acid deficiency.

Toxicity

Dr. Ernest Krebs, Jr., claims that pure pangamic acid is not harmful to humans. But, it can cause kidney damage in animals.

On the other hand, some contaminants commonly found in products sold as pangamic acid can cause damage. For example, diisopropyl amine can lower your blood pressure and body temperature. Dichloroacetate is mutagenic (causes basic changes in body cells), and 90 percent or more of all mutagenic compounds can cause cancer. Dimethylglycine has the potential of forming nitrosoamine, a cancer-causing chemical, in your stomach.

Therapeutic Uses

No therapeutic uses of pangamic acid have been verified.

Unsubstantiated Claims

Pangamic acid has been promoted for uses for which its value has not been proven. We cannot recommend that you take pangamic acid to treat: alcoholism, angina, asthma, atherosclerosis, autism, blood cholesterol, cancer, circulation diseases, headaches, hepatitis, hypertension, liver cirrhosis, multiple sclerosis, muscle injury, rheumatic fever, or rheumatism.

Availability

B_{15} has been banned from interstate commerce. Still, Calcium pangamate, the calcium salt of pangamic acid (the form in which this substance is usually sold) can be purchased in vitamin and health food stores in 50 mg. tablets.

B_{17} (Laetrile)

Laetrile is not a vitamin. It is not essential to life and is not associated with deficiency symptoms.

The laetrile story is as confusing as that of pangamic acid. The original material isolated by Ernest Krebs, Sr., from apricot kernels was amygdalin, which contains cyanide. Amygdalin is only one of many naturally occurring molecules with cyanide in their structure, yet only that molecule has been proposed as having a therapeutic effect on cancer. Other plant seeds that contain one form or another of cyanide are cherry, peach, plum, flax, guava, quince, and apple.

Laetrile is a synthetic product that is almost identical to amygdalin. For those who are interested, laetrile has a glucuronic acid molecule substituted for two molecules of glucose. Laetrile was named vitamin B_{17} by Krebs, who considered it essential to life.

Function

Laetrile has no known function in man, and there are therefore no daily requirements.

Dietary Sources

Amygdalin can be found in a number of foods we eat regularly, as listed in Table 22. Fortunately, we are able to inactivate any cyanide in the food by naturally occurring enzyme systems.

Table 22
Vitamin B_{17} (Laetrile) Content of Selected Foods

Food	Approximate Content (mg./3.5 oz.)
Almonds	15–30
Bean sprouts	2,000
Bitter almonds	4,200
Black-eyed peas	34
Buckwheat	340
Kidney beans	34
Navy beans	34
White lima beans (the kind available in the United States)	170
Black lima beans (available in Puerto Rico)	1,700

Deficiencies

There are no known deficiency symptoms for amygdalin.

Toxicity

Cyanide poisoning is a definite possibility with laetrile treatments. To date, thirty-seven people have died and seventeen more have been poisoned, mostly by eating apricot or other fruit kernels. One eleven-month-old infant died after accidentally swallowing between one and five laetrile tablets.

The chance of cyanide poisoning is increased if you eat one of the foods that contain beta glucosidase together with laetrile or with a fruit kernel. These foods are: fresh fruits, raw vegetables (lettuce, mushrooms, green peppers, and celery), and sweet almonds.

Symptoms of cyanide poisoning usually begin within one and a half to two hours after eating fruit pits or taking the laetrile, but may take longer to develop. The first symptoms are usually sudden and severe vomiting with stomach pains. Then the victim becomes extremely tired and dizzy. Breathing becomes very difficult, and the victim may turn blue because his body gradually loses its ability to utilize oxygen. Cyanide poisoning victims must be taken to a hospital as quickly as possible for treatment.

Other side effects of laetrile treatment are stomach bleeding, low blood pressure, vomiting, headache, diarrhea, fever, rash, and weakness.

Therapeutic Uses

No therapeutic uses of laetrile have been verified.

Unsubstantiated Claims

Cancer Treatment
Laetrile's proposed role in the treatment of cancer merits some discussion here. The theory is that cyanide, which can kill *any* living cell, is the magic bullet that selectively kills only cancer cells.

When laetrile is eaten and absorbed by normal cells, an enzyme called rhodonase inactivates the cyanide, rendering it harmless so it can be passed out of the body via the urine. This is a normal process that goes on in everyone if small amounts of cyanide are ingested.

According to proponents of laetrile treatment, cancer cells are deficient in rhodonase and are surrounded by another enzyme, called beta glucosidase. Beta glucosidase releases cyanide from the laetrile so it can kill the cancerous cells while normal cells remain unaffected.

Laetrile is usually used in combination with a special "metabolic antineoplastic diet." The basics of this diet are no meat, fish, or fowl, no dairy products, no animal protein, increased amounts of fruit and vegetables, pangamic acid, oral pancreas enzymes, vitamin E, and large doses of vitamin C. Ironically, vitamin C could actually increase the rate at which laetrile is broken down, increasing the chances of cyanide poisoning.

Careful studies by competent investigators have not verified that cancer cells are deficient in rhodonase and surrounded by beta glucosidase. Furthermore, evaluations of laetrile and amygdalin in the treatment of many animal cancers have not shown any benefit. Retrospective studies of groups of cancer patients given laetrile have also not shown any value to this treatment. In 1982, laetrile was tested by the National Cancer Institute of the National Institutes of Health and found to be of no value in the treatment of cancer. It has been outlawed by the Food and Drug Administration and cannot be sold in interstate commerce.

Availability

When available, laetrile tablets usually contain 500 mg. of the compound. However, the lack of a standard for making laetrile makes it very difficult to be sure of the laetrile content of any individual tablet. Laetrile should not be taken under any circumstances.

F (Essential Fatty Acids)

The essential fatty acids fit two of the criteria set forward for the definition of a vitamin: they are essential to human nutrition and are associated with deficiency symptoms. But they fail to qualify as vitamins because they are considered a macronutrient, that is, they are required in relatively large amounts. Vitamins, by definition, are needed only in small amounts.

There is no doubt that we all need fatty acids in our diet. The two most important ones are the unsaturated fatty acids, linoleic acid and linolenic acid. Another substance, arachadonic acid, had been considered an essential fatty acid until it was shown in 1956 that the body makes its own arachadonic acid from linoleic acid.

function

The essential fatty acids (EFAs) participate in many important body processes. Some of these are the manufacture of lecithin, which is a main source of choline (see p. 185), the manufacture of cholesterol in the body, blood clotting, the perception of pain, and maintenance of skin and hair. It has also been estimated that as much as 20 percent of the gray matter of our brains is made of fatty acids.

The EFAs are an integral part of every cell but are particularly important to the function of cells in the reproductive tract, in endocrine glands where hormones are made, and in the cells that line blood vessels.

Daily Requirements

It is generally accepted that fatty acids should provide about 2 percent of daily caloric intake. However, it is impossible to provide an absolute daily requirement for EFA since the requirement depends on individual dietary intake and the rate at which the EFAs are used.

Supplemental EFA are probably needed only by people who have been fed intravenously for several weeks and have depleted their internal supply; this supplementation is provided by giving intravenous fat emulsion preparations. Otherwise, dietary supplementation is preferable.

Dietary Sources

The best sources of EFAs are the oils (safflower, sunflower, corn, soy, sesame, cottonseed, peanut, etc.), nuts, margarine, wheat germ, olives, eggs, liver, some vegetables, and fish. Since requirements are so individual and so closely tied to calorie intake, it serves no function to use a table listing specific milligram contents of these foods.

Deficiencies

People, especially those who are hospitalized, or who are under extreme pressure and stress will use their EFA stores at a faster rate than others and may become deficient more easily.

Symptoms of Deficiency

People with EFA deficiency may develop dry and scaly skin, brittle hair and dandruff, and diarrhea. They may not heal properly and can lose their hair.

The symptoms are very similar to those revealed by experiments with animals. In one study, rats on a fat-free diet developed scaly skin, slowed growth, and loss of kidney function, but the addition of linoleic acid cured all of their problems. In another study, fatty acid deficiency was reported in mice, but interestingly, the animals remained normal until placed into a stressful situation; then they were unable to heal minor skin wounds, became sterile, and were intolerant to low doses of X rays.

EFA deficiency is diagnosed by assessing the ratios of different fatty acids in the blood. The test is called the "triene to tetraene ratio" and examines the ratio between oleic acid (a nonessential fatty acid) and linoleic acid. Normally the ratio should be less than 0.4 to 1. If the number is larger, it is assumed that there is not enough linoleic acid in the blood and a deficiency exists.

Toxicity

The only toxicities associated with EFAs have been observed in hospitalized patients being treated with intravenous fat emulsion products. If overused, the EFAs have caused fat deposits in the liver, breathing difficulties, some minor enlargement of liver or spleen, seizures, fever, and shock. These are unlikely to occur with oral EFA supplements.

Therapeutic Uses

EFA supplementation is widely used in hospitals to treat people being fed intravenously. Products containing soybean oil or safflower oil are used to provide calories and to satisfy the body's need for fatty acids.

Unsubstantiated Claims

EFAs have been promoted for other uses for which their value has not been proven. Although extensive research is being conducted into the role of EFAs and the possible need for EFA supplements, we cannot recommend, at this time, that you take EFAs to treat: acne, aging, allergy, arthritis, asthma, blood cholesterol, bronchitis, colitis, the common cold, constipation, diabetes, diarrhea, eczema, hair loss, heart disease, leg cramps, Meniere's disease, mental illness, multiple sclerosis, obesity, prostate disease, psoriasis, tooth and gum problems, or underweight.

Availability

EFAs, marketed as vitamin F, can be purchased in vitamin stores and health food outlets. Usually, these capsules contain linseed, safflower, sunflower or one of the other oils high in linoleic acid.

P (Bioflavinoids)

Bioflavinoids are yellow pigments found in a wide variety of plants. They cannot be considered vitamins because they have no established role in human nutrition and a dietary shortage of bioflavinoids does not produce deficiency symptoms.

Two bioflavinoids, rutin and hesperidin, have been called vitamin P.

Function

Bioflavinoids are claimed to have an action similar to vitamin C because they have a slight chemical similarity. Thus, they have been promoted as replacements for or supplements to be taken with vitamin C.

Daily Requirements

None have been established for the bioflavinoids.

Dietary Sources

The pulp and rind of citrus fruits and buckwheat leaves are sources of bioflavinoids.

Deficiencies

There are no known deficiency symptoms of bioflavinoids.

Toxicity

No toxicity is known.

Therapeutic Uses

No therapeutic uses of bioflavinoids have been verified.

Unsubstantiated Claims

Prevention of Bleeding
It is claimed that the bioflavinoids are useful in preventing bleeding caused by capillary fragility because they can supplement or duplicate the function of vitamin C. Vitamin C plays a role in maintaining the supportive structure in tissues surrounding the capillaries, the smallest blood vessels; deficiency leads to a collapse of these structures and therefore bleeding.

This claim for bioflavinoids is not supported by objective evidence.

Prevention and Cure of the Common Cold
Bioflavinoids are alleged to increase the efficiency of vitamin C in treating or preventing the common cold. This claim also has no objective backing.

Bioflavinoids have also been promoted for other uses for which their value has not been proven. We cannot recommend that you take bioflavinoids to treat: arteriosclerosis, arthritis, bleeding ulcers, blood cholesterol, bruises, hemorrhoids, hemophilia, hypertension, infections, inner ear disease, leukemia, pneumonia, pyorrhea, rheumatism, rheumatic fever, scurvy, skin problems, stroke, or varicose veins.

Availability

Citrus bioflavinoids can be purchased in vitamin centers or health food stores as 500 mg. tablets. Rutin tablets are available in strengths of 50 mg. and 100 mg. Tablets of rutin (50 mg.) plus vitamin C (300 mg.) are also sold in these outlets.

One of the most widely sold brands of bioflavinoids is called CVP (100 mg. capsules). The 200 mg. capsules of this product are called duo-CVP. Hesperidin complex is sold under the name of Hesper Capsules (100 mg.) and Hesper Bitabs (200 mg.).

Bioflavinoids are also included in some multivitamin formulas (Lipoflavinoid, some geriatric formulas, etc.).

Table 9

Vitamin Deficiency and Toxicity Symptoms

Vitamin	Best Sources	Deficiency Symptoms	Toxicity Symptoms
B₁ Thiamin	lean beef and pork, whole grains, enriched white flour, rice bran, soybeans, sunflower seeds, peanuts	*marginal deficiency:* loss of appetite, weight loss, nausea, vomiting, weakness, fatigue, nervous system problems such as rolling of eyeballs, depression, memory loss, difficulty in concentrating, personality changes *gross deficiency (beriberi):* muscle weakness, decreased reflex activity, fluid in arms and legs (edema), enlargement of heart, nausea and vomiting, nervous system problems similar to those of marginal deficiency	considered nontoxic
B₂ Riboflavin	lean beef and pork, chicken, milk, cheese, eggs, enriched white flour, spinach	*marginal deficiency:* red eyes, loss of facial color, sores at corner of mouth, sore throat, magenta coloration of tongue, red and raw lips, skin sores, greasy and scaly rash on face, rash in genital area *severe deficiency* is rare, but can cause anemia and nerve disease	considered nontoxic

Vitamin	Best Sources	Deficiency Symptoms	Toxicity Symptoms
B₃ Nicotinic Acid (Niacin)	lean beef, liver, turkey, tuna, whole grains, peanuts	*marginal deficiency:* diarrhea, headache, nervousness, swollen and red tongue	burning flush on face and hands, upset stomach, cramps, nausea, vomiting, diarrhea
		severe deficiency (pellagra): skin rash, cracking and bleeding skin, darkened areas of skin, diarrhea, red and swollen tongue, excess saliva, nausea, vomiting, mental disorientation, irritability, anxiety, hallucinations, delirium	severe toxicity can cause: liver damage, difficulty in metabolizing blood sugar, disturbed heart rhythm, rash over large areas, gouty arthritis
B₅ Pantothenic Acid	lobster, eggs, blue cheese, corn, peas, chickpeas, soybeans, sunflower seeds	*rare symptoms:* nausea, numbness in extremities, sleep disturbances, muscle spasms and cramps, poor muscle coordination, headache, fatigue, stomach pains, stomach gas, diarrhea, occasional vomiting	considered nontoxic

B₆ **Pyridoxine**	lean beef and pork, fish, eggs, whole grains, carrots, sunflower seeds	*rare symptoms:* irritability, confusion, nervousness, numbness of extremities, rash, sores on lips, tongue, and mouth, magenta coloration of tongue, seizures, anemia	generally nontoxic, but high doses can cause: nerve disorders, including difficulty in walking, numb hands difficult to control, loss of some sensory perceptions, including loss of feeling around mouth
B₁₂ **Cyanocobola-** **mine**	lean beef, liver, fish, shellfish, eggs, Camembert, blue cheese, Gorgonzola	*pernicious anemia:* loss of reflexes, nerve sensation, and function usually manifested in the form of tingling numbness in arms and legs, mood swings, memory losses, visual difficulties *megaloblastic anemia:* irritability, weakness, lack of energy, sleeping difficulties, loss of facial color	sudden stoppage of high doses results in deficiency symptoms considered nontoxic
Vitamin H **Biotin**	liver, butter, eggs, rice, peas, soybeans, sunflower seeds	*rare symptoms:* waxy appearance, nausea, loss of appetite, numbness, muscle pains, rash, loss of body hair, tiredness, depression, anemia, high blood cholesterol	considered nontoxic

Vitamin	Best Sources	Deficiency Symptoms	Toxicity Symptoms
Folic Acid	liver, barley, leafy green vegetables, beans, lentils, peanuts	*megaloblastic anemia*: irritability, weakness, lack of energy, sleeping difficulties, loss of facial color	considered nontoxic
Vitamin C Ascorbic Acid	broccoli, Brussels sprouts, spinach, green peppers, citrus fruit	*marginal deficiency*: shortness of breath, digestive difficulties, bleeding gums, easy bruising, swollen or painful joints, nosebleeds, anemia, susceptibility to infection, slow wound healing *severe deficiency (scurvy)*: loss of strength to point of inability to stand, shrunken black tendons, purple spots on skin, rotting gums, and loose teeth	generally nontoxic but can cause stomach upset and diarrhea megadoses can cause crystals to form in urinary tract, possibly leading to kidney stones, or to interference with elimination of uric acid, possibly leading to gout sudden stoppage of high doses results in deficiency symptoms
Vitamin A	liver, fish, shrimp, milk, butter, eggs, spinach, broccoli, carrots, endive, pumpkin, winter squash, cantaloupe, apricots	poor night vision, damage to cornea, dry, rough, or cracked skin, susceptibility to respiratory infection, hearing, taste, smell, and nerve damage, reduced sweat gland function.	vomiting, headache due to excess fluid in skull, symptoms of brain tumor, difficulty sleeping, joint pains, constipation, rough skin

Vitamin D	exposure to sunshine, liver, sardines, salmon, tuna, cod liver oil, fortified milk and margarine, eggs, mushrooms	*other possible effects:* slow growth, thickening of bones, kidney stones, diarrhea, reduced production of steroid hormones weakening the immune system, infant malformation	weakness, tiredness, headache, nausea, vomiting, loss of appetite, constipation or diarrhea, excessive thirst and urination, protein in urine, high blood pressure, high blood cholesterol, hardening of the arteries, mental retardation, slow growth, liver damage, and kidney failure
		rickets in children: bent, bowed legs, weak muscles, late tooth development	
Vitamin E	wheat germ, plant oils, margarine, cabbage, sunflower seeds, nuts	*rare symptoms:* anemia, fluid in arms and legs (edema)	generally nontoxic, but stomach upset, diarrhea, dizziness, and increased blood clotting time possible

Vitamin	Best Sources	Deficiency Symptoms	Toxicity Symptoms
Vitamin K	liver, oats, Cheddar cheese, Camembert cheese, Brussels sprouts, spinach, cabbage, turnip greens, cauliflower	rare except in newborn infants, but bleeding tendency possible	generally nontoxic, but a form of jaundice can occur in premature infants

Part III

MINERAL PROFILES

10

Essential Minerals

Calcium

Every schoolchild has heard that calcium is needed to build strong bones and teeth. What isn't often appreciated is the critical importance of this mineral in the blood and the body's complex mechanism for assuring that blood calcium levels remain constant at all times, even if bones must be weakened to supply necessary calcium.

Function

Calcium, together with phosphorous and magnesium, is a primary ingredient of bones, the skeletal framework that keeps us upright and mobile. More than 99 percent of the total store of calcium in your body is contained in bone, yet the remaining 1 percent plays a critical role in several other important functions. Calcium is essential to normal clotting of the blood, muscle contraction, heart function, nerve function, the storage and release of body hormones, and the utilization of amino acids as building blocks for all body proteins.

If you take in between 500 and 1,500 mg. of calcium every day, your body will take what it needs for daily function, send some to storage in the bone, and eliminate the rest through the urine. If average daily intake drops below these levels for any length of time, calcium will be withdrawn from bone to maintain body function.

The maintenance of proper blood calcium levels is controlled by a complex system involving vitamin D, parathyroid hormone, and calcitonin, a hormone produced by the thyroid gland. Vitamin D regulates the absorption of calcium from the gastrointestinal tract by activating the transport system responsible for moving calcium from the intestine into the blood. If blood calcium levels are low, vitamin D causes the kidney to excrete less calcium and stimulates the removal of calcium from bone. Vitamin D must be activated to perform this function, a role fulfilled by the parathyroid hormone. This hormone is also largely responsible for controlling the delicate balance between calcium and phosphorous levels in the blood; if calcium is very high, phosphorous will be excreted, and vice versa.

The final participant in calcium metabolism is calcitonin. Its function is the opposite of parathyroid hormone; it stops the movement of calcium out of the bone and into blood.

Daily Requirements

Unfortunately, the exact daily requirement of calcium is unknown, and the human body seems to be able to adapt to diets that provide as little as 300 mg. and as much as 1,500 mg. of calcium per day.

The average adult RDA for calcium is 800 mg. per day, to be increased to 1,200 mg. per day during pregnancy and breastfeeding. In addition, some experts have begun to promote the concept that this is not enough for older people, particularly older white women, who are at greater risk of developing osteoporosis, and have proposed that their daily calcium intake be raised to 1,000 mg.

Dietary Sources

We get most of our calcium from milk and milk products. Cheese and yogurt are particularly good sources because most of

Calcium Content of Selected Foods
Average adult RDA is 800 mg.

Food	Approximate Content (mg. per 3 oz.)
Almonds	214
Brazil nuts	171
Bread (whole wheat)	91
Dates (pitted)	53
Figs (dried)	114
Haddock (fried)	41
Milk	107
Carob	315
Caviar	252
Cheddar cheese	682
Eggs	49
Ice cream	112
Kelp	990
Molasses, light	150
Parmesan cheese	1,036
Prunes (dried)	80
Pistachio nuts	117
Raisins	56
Rhubarb	87
Salmon	135
Sardines	315
Seaweed	1,710
Sesame seeds	1,080
Soybeans	214
Sunflower seeds	108
Swiss cheese	841
Walnuts	85
Watercress	135
Yogurt	105

their calcium is found as highly concentrated calcium caseinate, a form of calcium the body finds particularly easy to use. Additional good sources are listed in the accompanying table. In this context, it should be emphasized that calcium can easily be obtained in a palatable form from food sources. Many of the calcium supplements are difficult for people to take simply because they do not taste good and may be difficult to swallow.

Deficiencies

With a system as complex as that involving calcium function, malfunction can occur at several points, and regulation of calcium in the body is a problem for many people. Difficulties with calcium levels in the blood are usually not caused by the amount of calcium taken in but are more likely to be associated with the regulatory hormones. People who make too much or too little parathyroid hormone or calcitonin, who don't take in or make enough vitamin D, or whose kidneys or livers cannot activate vitamin D may develop blood levels of calcium that are too low or too high.

High protein diets can also increase calcium loss because of the involvement of calcium in the body systems that break down proteins. In addition, the absorption of calcium from the intestine into the bloodstream may be interfered with if you eat foods such as rhubarb and spinach, which contain a chemical called oxalic acid, and dairy products with high levels of phosphate. Both oxalic acid and phosphate can interact with calcium in the stomach and prevent the latter from being absorbed into the bloodstream.

Some drugs, especially those used to treat epilepsy and other seizure disorders, speed the inactivation of vitamin D and can, therefore, lead to calcium deficiency. People taking phenytoin or another antiepileptic medication should consider modest supplements of vitamin D. Children taking one of these medicines should also be sure that their calcium intake is at least at the RDA level of 800–1,200 mg. per day.

Symptoms of Deficiency
When there is not enough calcium in the blood of growing children, they develop a disease known as rickets. In this disease, developing bones become deformed because they are too

weak to support the weight of a growing child. Rickets is rare in the United States and other developed countries because the necessity of calcium was recognized long ago. However, some Third World countries face a major problem in the area of child nutrition and rickets, with its characteristic sign of bowed legs.

In adults, low calcium intake can lead to osteomalacia, a disease in which bone is weakened because of the withdrawal of calcium, or osteoporosis, a condition in which there is a significant loss of bone mass and eventually leads to bone weakness and the inability of bone to bear the body's weight. This bone weakness makes its victims susceptible to fractures. The treatment of osteoporosis and osteomalacia are of major importance to older white women—the group which seems to be most susceptible to these diseases. While there is no cure as yet, several treatments have shown promise, including calcium supplements, small amounts of vitamin D (to assure that enough is present in the system), and low-dose estrogen replacement therapy.

Extremely low blood calcium can also cause muscle contractions, throat spasms, and convulsive seizures. These conditions require hospitalization and treatment with calcium, vitamin D, and other medications. Treatment of this problem can be very difficult if the basic difficulty lies with the calcium regulatory system.

Toxicity

Calcium is considered relatively nontoxic, but taking very large doses over an extended period of time can lead to the deposition of calcium in tissues throughout the body. One result of deposition of calcium in the kidneys can be the formation of calcium kidney stones.

Interactions

In addition to its relationship to phosphorous as discussed under "Functions," calcium can interact with zinc digitalis drugs taken for heart failure, antibiotic tetracycline, vitamin C and certain blood and urine tests. See Part IV, "Vitamin, Mineral, and Drug Interactions," for details.

Therapeutic Uses

Calcium supplements may be given to counteract any of the standard symptoms of calcium deficiency reviewed earlier in this profile. However, such symptoms will not be alleviated by calcium unless they are, in fact, caused by calcium deficiency.

In addition to prevention and alleviation of rickets in children and osteomalacia or osteoporosis in adults, calcium may also play an important role in the regulation of blood pressure. A recent study documented the fact that healthy men taking supplements of 1 g. of calcium per day experienced a 9 percent reduction in blood pressure within the first few weeks of calcium supplementation. Women experienced a decrease of about 5.5 percent. The conclusions of this study must be verified with more detailed studies, but the implications are that calcium supplementation may benefit people with high blood pressure.

A related group of drugs, the calcium or slow channel blockers, are being studied for their usefulness as blood pressure–lowering medicines. It is thought that they may be able to reduce pressure by slowing the movement of calcium out of the muscle cells that control the pressure in our blood vessels. If this is true, calcium supplements and drugs that affect calcium may also have this effect by raising muscle calcium levels. However, do not start using supplemental calcium to treat high blood pressure without consulting your doctor, and do not stop any high blood pressure medicines prescribed by your doctor.

Unsubstantiated Claims

Calcium has also been promoted for other uses for which its value has not been proven. We cannot recommend that you take calcium to treat: allergies, anemia, arthritis, cataracts, celiac disease, colitis, the common cold, constipation, diabetes, diarrhea, dizziness, epilepsy, fever, fractures, hardening of the arteries, hemorrhoids, hemophilia, leg cramps, insomnia, mental illness, Meniere's disease, nephritis, Parkinson's disease, tuberculosis, or worms.

Availability

Calcium is not taken in pure form but is always combined with other chemicals, or "salts." Therefore, calcium supplements are known as calcium salts. Different combinations, listed below, are available, and the amount of pure calcium in each form varies considerably. The important thing to remember is to measure the amount of calcium in the supplement, not the total amount of calcium salt.

Calcium Salt	Percentage Calcium
Calcium gluconate	9.0
Calcium lactate	13.0
Calcium carbonate	40.0
Calcium glubionate	6.5
Dibasic calcium phosphate dihydrate	23.0

If you take a gram of calcium gluconate, you will get only 90 mg. of calcium, while a gram of calcium carbonate (also known as chalk), provides 400 mg. When selecting the form of calcium you use for supplementation, the form with the larger percentage will provide the total amount of calcium in a smaller quantity.

Some people prefer to take their calcium as dolomite or bonemeal because of their tremendously high calcium count. Dolomite has almost 19 g. in 3 oz., and bonemeal has 36 g. in 3 oz. This concentration means that only small amounts of either form of calcium must be taken as a daily supplement.

However, some samples of these products have recently been found to be contaminated with potentially unsafe quantities of lead. Bonemeal is obtained as a by-product of meat processing, and it is possible that heavy metal contaminants in the diets of feed animals find their way into the animals' bone, which is then marketed in the form of bonemeal tablets. Dolomite is a mixture of calcium and magnesium mined from the ground and may contain traces of some of the heavy metals.

Both bonemeal and dolomite are good examples of the "natural is not always better" argument. A highly purified, chemically produced form of calcium is your best bet. Many popular products (Os-Cal and others) contain calcium, phosphorous, vitamin D, and other minerals. They have been widely used as calcium supplements because of their ability to provide these three important elements in bone metabolism.

Calcium injections are available for administration by doctors to people whose blood calcium levels are so low as to cause muscle spasm.

Phosphorous

Phosphorous is an essential ingredient of bone, second in importance only to calcium, and these two minerals act as barometers for each other to maintain a constant ratio. Every bone in the body contains calcium and phosphorous in a ratio of two to one, and interestingly, the same ratio is found in human breast milk.

function

More than 80 percent of the phosphorous in your body is located in bone, but the remainder that is found in other parts of the body is involved in virtually every important chemical reaction in your body.

It is involved in the body's utilization of fats, proteins and carbohydrates (sugar). Phosphorous combines with blood fats to form substances called phospholipids, which are part of the basic structure of cells. It also combines with proteins and amino acids to play an important role in the function of cells. Finally, phosphorous combines with an amino acid to assist in the generation of energy.

About 70 percent of our dietary phosphorous is absorbed in the intestine, and this absorption is aided by the presence of vitamin D. Unless a person is deficient, most of the absorbed phosphorous is eliminated by the kidneys into the urine. About 30 percent of our dietary phosphorous escapes absorption and is found in our stools, but this absorption increases automatically when a person is deficient.

Because of its importance, phosphate is under tight biological control, and the controls are nearly the same as discussed earlier for calcium. The primary controller of phosphorous levels is parathyroid hormone. This hormone, when secreted by the parathyroid gland, increases phosphorous elimination in the urine. This effect is different from the hormone's action on calcium, where it serves to decrease elimination. Thus, when blood calcium is high, phosphate is low, and the reverse is true. The hormone calcitonin also enhances excretion of phosphate in the urine.

Daily Requirements

The average adult RDA for phosphorous is 800 mg. Pregnant and breastfeeding women need 1,200 mg.

Phosphorous Content of Selected Foods
Average adult RDA is 800 mg.

Food	Approximate Content (mg. per 3 oz.)
Almonds	454
Barley	260
Bread, whole wheat	244
Bread, white enriched	90
Carob	72
Cheddar cheese	430
Cheese food, pasteurized process	679
Chicken	260
Eggs	180
Flounder	306
Ice cream	104
Lamb	190
Calf's Liver	432
Milk	84
Peaches (dried)	105
Peanuts	366
Peas	360
Pork	180
Potatoes	59
Pumpkin seeds	1,000
Rice	200
Sardines	520
Scallops	325
Soybeans	500
Sunflower seeds	756
Tuna	315
Turkey	188
Veal	207

Dietary Sources

Phosphorous is found in almost all foods because it is a critical part of all living things; it is also a component of many food additives and is to be found in soft drinks. Dairy products, meats, and fish are particularly rich sources, but the phosphorous in nuts, legumes, and grains is not well absorbed because it is tied up with insoluble, unabsorbable material. Additional good sources are listed in the accompanying table.

Most people take in more phosphorous than they need from dietary sources.

Deficiencies

Phosphorous deficiencies are relatively uncommon. However, long-term use of large amounts of antacids containing aluminum (aluminum hydroxide antacids) can hinder absorption of phosphorous. Doses of 1 oz. of aluminum hydroxide three times a day for a few weeks can adversely affect phosphate levels, so if you are in this situation it would be wise to take a phosphate supplement or increase the phosphate in your diet.

Symptoms of deficiency including bone pain, loss of appetite, weakness, and easily broken bones have been attributed to loss of phosphorous and failure to absorb dietary phosphate because of overzealous use of aluminum antacids.

Toxicity

Too much phosphorous in the blood can cause an increased calcium loss. This results in bone demineralization and a resulting bone weakness. Toxicity is rare except when the kidneys are diseased and are unable to remove the phosphate. In such cases, a low-phosphate diet and even aluminum hydroxide antacids are prescribed.

Interactions

For phosphorous interaction with calcium, see "Functions" above.

Therapeutic Uses

Phosphorous supplements may be given to counteract any of the standard symptoms of phosphorous deficiency reviewed earlier in this profile. However, such symptoms will not be alleviated unless they are, in fact, caused by mineral deficiency.

In addition, sodium phosphate is used in both oral and rectal forms as a saline-type laxative (Fleets enema, Fleet Phospho soda) to draw water into the intestines and thereby increase intestinal contractions. However, overuse of these products can cause phosphorous toxicity.

Unsubstantiated Claims

None.

Availability

The best phosphate supplement is probably dibasic calcium phosphate either with or without vitamin D (depending on your vitamin D status). We do not recommend bonemeal because some samples have been shown by the FDA to be contaminated with lead. Lead poisoning is more dangerous than a marginal phosphate deficiency. Dibasic calcium phosphate is pure and inexpensive and provides ample calcium as well as phosphate.

Magnesium

Popularly known as a basic ingredient of over-the-counter laxatives, magnesium is, in fact, one of the three important "bone minerals," along with calcium and phosphorous.

Function

Over half the body's magnesium is found in bone. The remainder performs essential, though less familiar roles.

Magnesium is involved in the flow of elements across cell membranes, and here its most important function relates to muscle relaxation. Movement of calcium across cell membranes causes muscle contractions; when calcium leaves and is replaced by magnesium, muscles relax. Magnesium is also an essential part of the mechanism that transmits nerve impulses across cell membranes.

In addition, magnesium works with enzymes in breaking down sugar that has been stored in the liver from glycogen to glucose, the form in which it can be used for energy. This function is specifically related to magnesium's involvement in the transfer of energy via the movement of phosphate molecules.

Daily Requirements

The average adult RDA for magnesium is 325 mg. Pregnant and breastfeeding women need 450 mg.

Dietary Sources

Rich sources of magnesium include molasses, nuts, fish, and whole grains. Additional good sources are listed in the accompanying table.

Magnesium Content of Selected Foods

Average adult RDA is 325 mg.

Food	Approximate Content (mg. per 3 oz.)
Almonds	242
Barley	50
Beans, canned	33
Bluefish	220
Bread, white	23
Bread, whole wheat	41
Carp	230
Cod	176
Cornmeal	92
Crab (steamed)	159
Figs (dried)	64
Flounder	177
Haddock	179
Halibut	191
Hazelnuts	135

Food	Approximate Content (mg per 3 oz.)
Herring (fresh)	232
Lobster	166
Mackerel	217
Molasses, blackstrap	370
Oat cereal, dry	101
Oatmeal	130
Oats	125
Ocean perch	192
Oysters	130
Peanuts	185
Pike	194
Pistachios	145
Prunes (dried)	37
Raisins	32
Rice	108
Salmon	170
Scallops	189
Shad	236
Shrimp	199
Snails	225
Snapper	195
Soybeans	215
Spinach	52
Sunflower seeds	315
Swordfish	177
Tuna	75
Wheat germ	290
Yellow perch	163

Surveys of "typical" diets have shown that our intake is somewhat lower, at 180–300 mg., than the average RDA of 325 mg. for adults, without evidence of adverse effects.

Deficiencies

Because of the importance of magnesium to daily life, the body has become very efficient at conserving this mineral. Magnesium is excreted by the kidney, and when there is a shortage, excretion is sharply reduced. Absorption from the gut is also increased when the body is depleted. For these reasons, a deficiency is very rare. Deficiencies have, however, been observed in individuals with alcoholism, diabetes, chronic diarrhea, or damaged kidneys and in those fed intravenously without magnesium supplements.

Symptoms of deficiency include muscle contraction, convulsions, tremors, confusion, and delirium.

Toxicity

Toxicity is rare except in cases of kidney failure where excess magnesium is not eliminated from the body. Toxic signs of magnesium excess are muscle weakness, fatigue, low blood pressure, confusion, loss of reflexes, and depression of respiration and heart rate leading to death at very high magnesium levels. Toxicity with oral doses of magnesium preparations is uncommon because, as discussed in "Therapeutic Uses," it serves as a laxative. The diarrhea resulting from too large an intake of magnesium would rid the body of an excess.

Interactions

Magnesium can interact with drugs used to relax muscles during surgery, oral anticoagulant drugs, and the tranquilizer chlorpromazine (Thorazine). See Part IV, "Vitamin, Mineral, and Drug Interactions."

Therapeutic Uses

Magnesium supplements may be given to counteract any of the standard symptoms of magnesium deficiency reviewed earlier in this profile. However, such symptoms will not be alleviated by magnesium unless they are, in fact, caused by mineral deficiency.

Magnesium is also frequently used as a laxative. Magnesium sulfate (Epsom salts), magnesium hydroxide (milk of magnesia, Haley's M-O), and magnesium citrate are so-called saline-type laxatives that draw fluid from the tissues and serum into the intestine. The result is stimulation of the intestine to contract. In this process up to 20 percent of the magnesium in these products may be absorbed, but ordinarily this causes no problem because the kidney excretes it into the urine. However, people who overuse such laxatives over long periods of time or who have kidney failure may develop magnesium toxicity.

Another therapeutic use of magnesium results from its depressing effects on muscles. Injections of magnesium sulfate are sometimes used to block the seizures that occur with the toxemia of pregnancy.

Unsubstantiated Claims

None.

Availability

Magnesium sulfate, magnesium gluconate, and a magnesium-protein complex are available for oral use. Injectable magnesium sulfate products are also available. Dolomite, a magnesium and calcium carbonate complex mined from the ground, is used by some as a source of magnesium. As in the case of calcium, the FDA has found lead contamination in some of this material, and we therefore do not recommend it.

Iodine

Well known as an antiseptic for cuts, iodine is actually much more important for its role in the proper functioning of the thyroid gland in the neck, the regulator of body metabolism. Insufficient iodine in the diet results in an underactive thyroid or in goiter, a condition in which the thyroid becomes tremendously enlarged in an effort to compensate for lack of iodine.

Goiter was once very prevalent in the Midwest because of the low iodine content of locally produced foods—inland soils are very low in iodine. But nowadays several factors combine to minimize the incidence of goiter everywhere, in spite of iodine-poor regional soils.

Most important is the use of iodized salt. Although the addition of iodine to salt is voluntary in the United States—in contrast to some countries, where it is required by law—most table salt consumed here is iodized, and all such products are clearly labeled. In addition, livestock used for meat is encouraged to lick salt blocks that contain iodine, thus increasing the iodine content of meat in our diets. Some fertilizers applied to soils also have added iodine, which in turn finds its way into plants that we eat.

Function

Over 80 percent of the iodine in the human body can be found in the thyroid gland, and without iodine all thyroid hormone production would come to a halt; iodine is responsible for the synthesis of thyroxine and diiodothyronine, the two important hormones produced by the thyroid. Since thyroid hormones are the "gas pedal" for your body's metabolism, the rate of metabolism and the heat produced by the body is directly affected by them. Low thyroid levels result in lassitude, listlessness, and generally sluggish behavior, whereas an abnormally high thyroid output is characterized by nervousness and hyperactivity.

Daily Requirements

The needs for iodine are considered to be met by intakes in the range of 100–200 mcg. per day; goiter is prevented by 50–70 mcg. The RDA value for iodine for adults is 150 mcg. per day, to be increased to 175 mcg. during pregnancy and 200 mcg. during lactation.

Dietary Sources

Seafood and plants grown near the sea are the richest sources of iodine. Milk is also high because dairy cattle lick salt blocks with iodine. Additional good sources are listed in the accompanying table.

Deficiencies

Severe childhood iodine deficiencies resulting in failure to make adequate amounts of thyroid hormone can cause depressed growth and delayed sexual development, mental retardation and

Iodine Content of Selected Foods
Average adult RDA is 150 mcg.

Food	Approximate Content (mcg. per 3 oz.)
Cantaloupe	18.0
Cod	126.0
Cod liver oil	755.0
Crab	28.0
Haddock	280.0
Halibut, broiled	41.4
Herring	47.0
Lobster	90.0
Oysters	44.0
Salmon, canned	46.0
Salt, sea	85.0
Salt, table (with iodine)	9,000.0
Sardines, canned	33.0
Seaweed	55,800.0
Shrimp, boiled	117.0
Sunflower seeds	63.0
Tuna, canned	14.0
Turnip greens	42.0

deafness. Cretinism, which develops in an infant after severe iodine deficiency during pregnancy, is a combination of dwarfishness and feeblemindedness.

Goiter is, of course, the classic deficiency disease in adults. It is usually caused by insufficient iodine but can also result from the consumption of large quantities of raw foods containing substances called goitrogens. These are chemicals that inhibit thyroid hormone synthesis. The condition is worsened when iodine intake is low and may be relieved by taking iodine supplements. Goitrogens are present in such vegetables as spinach, lettuce, turnips, beets, rutabaga, kale, and casava but are destroyed in cooking. Goitrogen-induced goiter is rare because these vegetables generally are not eaten in huge quantities.

As a whole, we are getting plenty of iodine in our diets and there is no need to be concerned about deficiency, provided that you are using iodized salt, are not eating huge amounts of goitrogenic vegetables, and do not have an underactive thyroid. There is generally no reason to take iodine supplements.

Toxicity

Doses of iodine under about 3,000 mcg. per day are considered nontoxic but can cause rash, headache, difficulty in breathing due to fluid in the lungs, and a metallic taste in the mouth.

Paradoxically, very high iodine intake (over 20,000 mcg. a day) can cause a form of goiter known as "iodine goiter." This is because excessive quantities of iodine can actually inhibit the release of thyroid hormone from the thyroid gland and result in symptoms very similar to those of iodine deficiency. "Iodine goiter" is known in certain parts of Japan where substantial quantities of seaweed are consumed as a food staple and iodine intakes can be as high as 50,000–80,000 mcg. per day.

There is a general upward trend in the iodine content of most diets due to the overuse of iodized salt, the use of iodine-containing antiseptics on dairy farms, traces of which get into the milk, and the use of iodine-containing compounds as bread dough conditioners in the baking industry. While some people are concerned about this upward trend, average consumption is still far less than would be expected to cause any signs of toxicity.

Interactions

Iodine can interact with lithium carbonate taken for manic depressive illness and can interfere with certain blood and urine tests. See Part IV, "Vitamin, Mineral, and Drug Interactions."

Therapeutic Uses

Iodine supplements may be given to counteract the standard symptoms of iodine deficiency reviewed earlier in this profile. However, such symptoms will not be alleviated by iodine unless they are, in fact, caused by mineral deficiency.

In addition to treating underactive thyroid and goiter, iodine supplements may also be given to reduce thyroid function in people with overactive thyroid glands prior to surgery. This is done to inactivate the gland temporarily until the surgery can be performed and the problem cured permanently.

Aside from thyroid function, iodine is widely used as a medical antiseptic. Iodine complexes that release their mineral content slowly, such as povidone iodine, are superior for this purpose over plain solutions of iodine, such as tincture of iodine, because they work for a longer period of time. However, in either form, the antiseptic effect produced by iodine is quite effective against virtually all bacteria. An iodine concentration of 1 percent is required for the mineral to be antiseptic.

The antiseptic property of iodine is also responsible for its use as a water "sanitizer." By adding small amounts of iodine to the water, any offending bacteria present will be killed and the water made safe to drink. Adding three drops of tincture of iodine to a quart of water will render the water safe to drink in fifteen minutes without ruining the taste of the water.

Unsubstantiated Claims

Iodine has also been promoted for a variety of other uses for which its value has not been proven. Therefore we cannot recommend that you take this mineral to treat: angina pectoris, arteriosclerosis, or arthritis. It will also not solve any hair problems or restore lost vim and vigor.

Availability

Potassium iodide tablets in strengths of 50–300 mg. are available, as is a highly concentrated solution containing 5 g. per teaspoon, which is prescribed in doses of several drops.

Iron

Iron, which is so essential to healthy blood, is the one mineral in which large segments of the population of the United States are chronically deficient.

Menstruating women are the largest category, and surveys have shown iron deficits in 10–30 percent of those studied.

Deficiencies in pregnant women range from 10–60 percent, and infants from two months to two years of age are also at risk.

To combat this problem, "enriched" flours have been fortified with iron for some time, and in 1975 the amount of iron to be added was ordered increased. Currently there is considerable interest in additional government regulation to require the fortification of more foods with iron.

Function

Of the iron in the body, 60–70 percent is stored in hemoglobin, the red part of red blood cells. Hemoglobin performs the vital function of carrying oxygen from lungs to body tissues.

Hemoglobin is also a component of myoglobin, an iron protein complex in muscles. This complex helps muscles get extra energy when they are hard at work.

In addition, iron is important to the function of many enzymes involved in the production of energy.

Iron is stored in the liver, spleen, and bone marrow.

Daily Requirements

The RDA is 10 mg. for adult males and 18 mg. for adult females.

Dietary Sources

Liver is the richest source of iron. Egg yolks, other meats, whole grain products, nuts, and seafood also contain substantial amounts, and wine contains some. Additional good sources are listed in the accompanying table.

Iron Content of Selected Foods

Average adult RDA is 10 mg. for men, 18 mg. for women.

Food	Approximate Content (mg. per 3 oz.)
Bacon	3.0
Beef	3.0
Bonemeal	74.0
Bread, white, enriched	2.3

Essential Minerals

Food	Approximate Content (mg per 3 oz.)
Bread, whole wheat	2.3
Cashews	3.5
Carrots, raw	0.6
Caviar	10.8
Cheddar cheese	0.9
Chicken	1.5
Chickpeas	6.2
Currants, black	1.0
Eggs	2.0
Egg yolks	
Figs, fried	3.2
Green beans	1.4
Haddock	1.0
Lentils	6.0
Calf's liver	8.0
Loganberries	1.0
Lychees	1.5
Milk, whole	0.0
Molasses, blackstrap	8.1
Mussels	5.3
Oysters, canned	5.0
Peanut butter	1.8
Pecans	2.2
Pistachios	6.5
Pears (dried)	1.1
Persimmons (native)	2.25
Pork	2.7
Prunes (dried)	3.2
Pumpkin seeds	10.0
Raisins	3.2
Seaweed	81.0
Sesame seeds	9.0
Snails	3.2
Spinach	3.0
Veal	2.9
Walnuts	5.4
Wheat germ	8.5

Unfortunately, iron-rich foods are not as much of a help as one might think because our iron absorption from foods is very poor. It has been estimated that, on an average, only about 10 percent of food iron is absorbed, although this can increase to 20 percent if the body's iron stores are low. However, these figures are only gross estimates and an oversimplification. In fact, the amount of iron absorbed depends on quite a number of factors. One major consideration is the nature of the iron in the food. Iron that is bound to hemoglobin, as would be available in red meats and liver, is easily absorbed, and as much as 20–30 percent may be available for absorption. Iron not bound to hemoglobin (so-called inorganic iron) is poorly absorbed. The inorganic iron found in the plants, for example, is only absorbed to the extent of about 5 percent.

Compounding the complexity of calculating the amount of iron that is available in foods is the fact that other food substances can influence the amount of iron absorbed. For example, nutritionists speak of "highly available" and "poorly available" meals with respect to iron. Including meat in a meal will substantially increase the absorption of the inorganic iron found in vegetables; 200 mg. of vitamin C will increase absorption of inorganic iron by as much as 25–50 percent. On the other hand, absorption is decreased by tea, antacids, tofu and other soy proteins and the tetracycline antibiotics.

The iron content of foods, especially acidic foods, can be dramatically increased by preparation in iron cookware. The iron content of spaghetti sauce, for example, increases from 2.7 mg. per ounce to about 80 mg. per ounce if prepared in a cast iron container.

Deficiencies

The disease associated with iron deficiency is hypochromic (light in color), microcytic (small red blood cell) anemia. The red blood cells become smaller than normal and pale in color due to the lack of iron in the hemoglobin. Symptoms of deficiency are related to poor oxygen delivery to tissues and include listlessness, heart palpitations upon exertion, fatigue, irritability, a general pale appearance, cracking of the lips and tongue, difficulty in swallowing, and a general feeling of poor health.

Deficiencies can be determined by examining the blood to look at the intensity of color of red blood cells or by measuring the volume of red blood cells compared with the total volume of blood spun at high speed (the hematocrit test). Other tests involve measuring the content of iron protein complexes in blood and bone marrow.

A true iron deficiency anemia responds fairly rapidly to iron supplementation, but the supplementation should be continued for a time (months) to replenish the iron stores in the body. It is important to remember, however, that anemia can be a symptom of other deficiencies, or even of more serious illnesses. It can result from a folic acid deficiency or a vitamin B_{12} deficiency as well as from an iron deficiency. Anemia can also be caused by an adverse reaction to drugs or toxins in the environment. Any bleeding from ulcers or cancer would give the outward appearance of a simple iron deficiency anemia. Although consumption of iron products may relieve some of the symptoms of the disease, it will not cure the disease. You should consult your physician to determine the cause of anemia since it could be related to internal bleedings, rather than try to treat it yourself. A delay in treatment could have serious consequences.

Iron and Menstruating Women

During menstruation, blood loss accounts for substantial iron losses. The average menstruating female loses, on a daily basis, about 0.7 mg. of iron, but this value is highly variable among women because of substantial differences in the blood loss during menstruation. A woman who has a heavy menstrual flow may lose as much as 2 mg. of iron on a daily basis. Working though with the average figure, we have an inherent loss of 1 mg. and a loss during menstruation of 0.7 mg., giving us a total average daily loss for menstruating females of 1.7 mg. If we assume that 10 percent of the iron consumed is available, then this average woman would need to take in 17 mg. of iron per day, and this is why the RDA for women is set at 18 mg. Unfortunately, the "average" 2,100-calorie diet provides only about 13 mg. of iron, and thus this "average" woman eating an average diet would be expected to show some signs of iron deficiency.

If you are in this category, you should modify your diet to

increase iron intake and to include items that would enhance iron absorption. The easiest way to do this is to make sure that you eat some meat and/or vitamin C–containing fruit every day. Alternatively, an iron supplement may be warranted.

Iron and Pregnant Women

Pregnancy creates a tremendous strain on iron stores. A developing fetus needs plenty of iron, and the blood volume of the mother is substantially increased during pregnancy, which further increases the need for iron. The demand for iron is such that the daily requirement may be close to 6 mg. per day, which translates to 60 mg. of dietary iron needed. Because it is almost impossible to get this much iron conveniently from food, pregnant women need to take iron supplements, and it is suggested that they continue to take supplements for two to three months after childbirth to compensate for the stores depleted during pregnancy.

Iron needs during lactation are not substantially different from those of nonpregnant women. While some iron is lost in the breast milk, this is compensated to some extent by the decrease in menstrual blood flow during breastfeeding.

Iron and Infants

If the mother is well nourished, the infant at birth should have ample iron, but after that there may be problems. Unfortunately, milk is not a very good source of iron, nor are the cereals and other baby foods that are consumed during the first two years of life. Breast milk has a small amount of iron but it is well absorbed by the breastfed infant. This puts the infant at risk of developing iron deficiencies because growing children need almost as much iron as do adults.

Many nutritionists now feel that iron supplements should be given to children during the first two years of life. Baby formulas are available with and without iron, and infant vitamin preparations are also available with and without iron. We suggest that infants be checked for iron deficiency. In many cases, supplements should be used.

Iron and Vegetarians

A vegetarian needs to be concerned about iron nutrition, but ample iron can be absorbed if enough vitamin C is taken with iron rich foods. Two recent surveys of vegetarians have failed to reveal any problems with iron nutrition in this population despite concern from a theoretical basis.

Toxicity

Doses of iron over 1,000 mg. can cause iron toxicity. Symptoms include vomiting, diarrhea, weak pulse, exhaustion, and stomach cramps. If the amount of iron ingested is high enough, one may go into a coma with cardiovascular collapse and death.

Ingestion of iron tablets is a frequent cause of poisoning in children because iron supplement tablets are attractive in appearance and are mistakenly taken as candy. They should be locked in a medicine cabinet.

Interactions

Iron can interact with allopurinol taken for gout, antacids, the antibiotics chloramphenicol (Chloromycetin) and tetracycline drugs, cholestyramine resin (Questran) for high blood cholesterol, pancreatic extract (pancreatin) for enzyme replacement, penicillamine (Cuprimine, Depen) for rheumatoid arthritis, vitamin C, vitamin E, calcium, copper, zinc, and claystarch (also interferes with iron absorption). See Part IV, "Vitamin, Mineral, and Drug Interactions."

Unsubstantiated Claims

None.

Availability

Ferrous sulfate tablets are inexpensive, and four 320 mg. tablets will provide between 25 and 50 mg. of absorbed iron. For most people, ferrous sulfate taken three to four times a day is more than adequate and there are no real advantages for the other more expensive products.

Sustained release or timed release products should be avoided because they deliver the iron to the lower reaches of the intestine, where it is less efficiently absorbed. Those would only be indicated if a person is having trouble with stomach irritation caused by the iron. Iron also tends to be constipating, and some products contain a stool softener to minimize this problem.

Since vitamin C increases the amount of iron absorbed, it is included in many iron-containing products. Between 200 and 400 mg. of vitamin C is needed to get the best absorption.

Zinc

Interest in zinc as a dietary supplement and nutritional agent has intensified over the last decade since reports of zinc deficiency syndromes have appeared in the medical literature. There also is contemporary interest in zinc because Western populations seem to have marginally low intakes, and inadequate zinc has been associated with poor healing and slow growth rates in children.

Function

Zinc is an essential feature of more than seventy enzymes. The most critical role that it plays in the body is in the synthesis of DNA and RNA, needed for cell division, cell repair, and cell growth. It also plays a crucial role in bone growth and development and aiding in normal reproductive function. In addition, zinc seems to be involved with activation of vitamin A in the eye and is thus a factor in night vision.

Daily Requirements

The RDA value is 15 mg., to be increased to 20 mg. during pregnancy and 25 mg. during lactation.

Most diets are marginally low in zinc, supplying 10–15 mg., and do not come close to supplying the zinc estimated to be required during pregnancy and lactation. For this reason, women should select a prenatal vitamin-mineral preparation that contains zinc—not all do.

Dietary Sources

Since zinc is so important to life processes, it is present in almost all living systems, but it is richest in meats, poultry, liver, eggs, seafood (especially oysters), and whole grains. Other good sources are listed in the accompanying table.

Zinc Content of Selected Foods

Average adult RDA is 15 mg.

Food	Approximate Content (mg. per 3 oz.)
Bacon	4.5
Barley	2.5
Beef	2.7
Beets	2.5
Bonemeal	3.3
Bread, white	1.0
Bread, whole wheat	2.5
Brewer's yeast	3.5
Cheddar cheese	0.8
Chicken	4.4
Cocoa	4.4
Coconut	2.7
Corn	2.8
Eggs	1.2
Herring	100.0
Lamb	4.8
Maple syrup	6.8
Molasses, blackstrap	7.2
Oysters	145.0
Pork	3.1
Sesame seeds	9.0
Soybeans	6.3
Sunflower seeds	5.9
Turkey	12.5
Walnuts	2.5
Wheat	2.9
Wheat germ	12.5
Yeast	9.0

However, our ability to absorb zinc from these foods is not uniform. The situation is similar to that discussed in the profile on iron in that the richest and best-absorbed source of zinc is meat products. The amount of zinc we take in from other good food sources depends on many factors, including certain combinations of foods and interaction of body chemicals. Do not take zinc supplements together with coffee, brown bread, dairy products, especially milk, cheese, or other high-calcium foods.

Another important consideration in evaluating dietary sources is the fact that refined food and the milling process to produce white flour remove most of the zinc content; whole wheat flour has six times as much zinc as white flour. So-called enriched bread and flour is only enriched in a very few specific vitamins and iron.

A varied diet including substantial amounts of raw vegetables and whole grain products is the best way to ensure that your zinc needs are met. Variety is important because heavy reliance on any single item for zinc, for example, high-fiber grains, may actually decrease the absorption of zinc, as discussed in the next section.

Deficiencies

Zinc deficiency in man was first noted during the 1960s in Egypt and other parts of the Middle East. The deficiency developed because of the use of unleavened whole wheat bread as a staple in the diet. Phytic acid, found in whole wheat flour, forms an insoluble complex with zinc, making it unavailable for absorption from the gastrointestinal tract. The symptoms seen in the Middle Eastern boys who were the subjects of this study were slowed growth, loss of appetite, loss of taste sensation, diarrhea, skin rash, slowed sexual (gonadal) development, and enlargement of the spleen and liver.

Another disease, called acrodermatitis enteropathica, is associated with the inability to absorb zinc efficiently from the gastrointestinal tract. People with this disease show the following symptoms: diarrhea, muscle wasting, hair loss, and skin lesions.

Zinc levels seem to fall, also, during stress, trauma, infectious diseases, and when large doses of steroid drugs are administered. Alcohol, even in moderate amounts, can increase the amount of zinc loss from the body in the urine and can impair the body's ability to combine zinc into its proper enzyme combinations in the liver. In addition, excessive intake of copper can increase an existing zinc deficiency.

Zinc deficiency may be diagnosed by clinical signs or by blood concentration. An enzyme in the blood called alkaline phosphatase is dependent upon zinc for activity and can also be used as an index of zinc nutrition. Each test has its drawbacks, and there is therefore disagreement over which produces the most accurate results.

Zinc and Pregnant Women

Women taking oral contraceptives develop low blood levels of zinc because of the action of the contraceptive hormones. Low zinc levels are also observed during pregnancy, probably due to similar hormone changes, although the fetus certainly draws heavily on the mother's zinc supply. Zinc intake in most pregnant women is only two-thirds of the RDA value. While the consequences of this are not clear, it is worrisome because animal studies have shown that zinc deficiencies can result in birth defects in the newborn and in low-birthweight infants.

Zinc and Vegetarians

Although some nutritionists have expressed concern that vegetarian diets might not provide enough zinc, recent surveys conducted on vegetarian volunteers have indicated that zinc levels seem to be adequate in these individuals. Soybean products that are used by vegetarians as a protein source may be a factor in supplying zinc and enhancing absorption.

Toxicity

Zinc can have some adverse effects, although it is not as toxic as some elements. Doses of more than 200 mg. have caused vomiting in adults, and higher doses can cause dehydration, stomach pains, poor muscle coordination, tiredness, and kidney failure. Supplements should be taken only for short intervals of time for a specific purpose.

Interactions

High zinc intakes can decrease absorption of iron and copper, and this could potentially lead to problems. Calcium interferes with zinc absorption. One group of investigators claims that high body zinc levels relative to body copper levels predisposes one toward coronary heart diseases, but this hypothesis is not universally accepted.

Therapeutic Uses

Zinc supplements may be given to counteract any of the standard symptoms of zinc deficiency reviewed earlier in this profile. However, such symptoms will not be alleviated by zinc unless they are, in fact, caused by mineral deficiency.

Zinc oxide applied to the skin has also been used for a long time to help in the healing of burns and other wounds and seems to be of some benefit.

Recent studies evaluating effects of zinc supplements on the speed of healing of surgical wounds and leg ulcers have revealed that zinc seems to play a role in the latter stages of wound healing, that is, after about ten days. Other studies have shown that in hospitalized patients who are marginally zinc deficient, extra zinc helps speed the rate of wound healing and restores sense of taste. The doses used to supplement these patients were high; they took about 220 mg. of zinc sulfate three times a day, which provides about 130 mg. of zinc. In most studies the only patients who realized substantial benefit from the zinc supplements were those who had been zinc deficient to begin with. Zinc in doses less than 200 mg. is harmless when taken for short periods of time (e.g. one to two months), and it may be that supplements can be of some benefit to stimulate healing after surgery, broken bones, wounds, etc. Some physicians are now starting to prescribe zinc for this purpose.

Unsubstantiated Claims

Zinc supplements have been used for arthritis and in patients with various cancers, but the evidence for improvement of their disease is not strong.

Availability

Zinc supplements are available as zinc sulfate tablets and capsules in strengths from 60 to 200 mg. and as zinc gluconate tablets in strengths of 35–200 mg. Zinc is also included in many vitamin-mineral preparations.

11

Important Trace Minerals

Chromium

Chromium is clearly essential in human nutrition, but the exact form of chromium that is used by the body is uncertain. Our diets seem to be marginally low in this element, and it is possible that supplements may help some diabetics.

Function

The best-studied feature of chromium is its effect on glucose metabolism. The body needs the hormone insulin to get glucose from the blood into tissues where it can be used to generate energy, and it is believed that chromium increases the sensitivity of tissues to the action of insulin. In a chromium-deficient state, increasing amounts of insulin are needed to maintain normal glucose utilization. Chromium itself has no effect on glucose; it only works together with insulin to drive sugar from blood to tissue.

Daily Requirements

There is no RDA for chromium. An estimated range considered "safe and adequate" for adults is 50–200 mg. The more carbohydrate you eat, the more chromium you need, but precise amounts are not known.

Dietary Sources

Accurate information on the chromium content of many common foods is lacking, and less than 1 percent of dietary chromium is absorbed. Oysters, eggs, whole grains, and yeast are considered good sources. Brewer's yeast provides approximately 70 mcg. per ounce and is the richest single source of chromium. Wine and beer also contain about 0.3 mcg. per 3 oz. Refining and processing of foods causes appreciable chromium loss.

Typical American diets seem to provide 50–80 mg. of chromium, and this is thought by some to be marginally low. Japanese diets provide 100–200 mg. per day.

Deficiencies

In animals, chromium deficiency has only been produced under experimental conditions. Symptoms are disturbances in glucose, fat, and protein metabolism as well as decreased growth rates and longevity. Chromium deficiency, resulting in disturbances of glucose, fat, and protein metabolism, has also been reported in people receiving long-term intravenous nutrition without protein supplementation. Additional evidence for human deficiencies comes from studies of patients with maturity-onset diabetes, as discussed under "Therapeutic Uses."

Toxicity

Chromium is considered to be relatively nontoxic in doses less than 1,000 mg. Chronic exposure to chromium dust in an industrial environment has been associated with an increase in lung cancer.

Therapeutic Uses

Investigations have shown that some maturity-onset diabetics can decrease their insulin requirements and improve glucose tolerance by taking chromium supplements.

Body chromium levels decrease with age, while glucose tolerance time (the length of time the body takes to utilize glucose) increases with age. An increased glucose tolerance test time can be a forerunner of diabetes, and reliable studies have shown that chromium supplementation is beneficial to some patients who have abnormalities in glucose metabolism. Usually 180–1,000 mg. of chromium trichloride are used, and supplementation must continue for months before an effect is observed. The implication of these studies is that the people who benefited were taking in too little chromium. At present, it is not known to what extent all types of diabetics would benefit from chromium supplements.

Chromium supplementation should only be undertaken under the care of a physician because wide swings in blood glucose concentrations should be avoided. Nevertheless, chromium supplements may be helpful for some. But it should never be used as the sole treatment for diabetes.

At present there are no therapeutic uses for chromium other than for glucose abnormalities.

Unsubstantiated Claims

None.

Availability

Chromium chloride is available by prescription in a solution for use in intravenous nutrition and without prescription in tablet and capsule form for oral supplementation. In our opinion, the dose should be kept below 1,000 mg. per day.

Copper

Copper is receiving special attention in research laboratories nowadays because some people are concerned that our copper intakes are inadequate and believe that copper supplements might help prevent heart diseases. Others point to dietary surveys over the past twenty years that show that we are taking in plenty of copper and that there are no signs of deficiency.

Function

Copper is a component of an enzyme called superoxide dismutase, which is involved in the regulation of oxygen level in body tissues. Excess oxygen can result in toxicity, which in turn results in destruction of body tissues. Superoxide dismutase prevents this by using up excess oxygen molecules.

In addition, copper is a major component of ceruloplasmin, which is essential for the transport of iron in the blood. Copper also affects the release of iron from the intestines into the blood and is needed for recycling of iron released from red blood cells that are dead.

Finally, in a more minor role, copper participates in the maintenance of body structure. In this capacity it is involved in linking collagen—the material that provides structure to soft tissues—with connective tissues.

Copper functions on a see-saw basis with molybdenum. If you have excess copper, your molybdenum level will drop; if you have excess molybdenum, your copper level will drop.

Daily Requirements

The adult requirements for copper are estimated to be 2–3 mg. The Food and Nutrition Board of the National Academy of Sciences does not list RDA values for copper, but the U.S. RDA value for adults and children four or more years of age is 2 mg.

Dietary Sources

Shellfish and organ meats are the richest sources of copper, but fish and nonleafy vegetables also provide ample copper. Additional good sources are listed in the accompanying table.

Refining and milling of foods and grains removes most of the mineral content. Therefore, the copper content of highly refined flours is low. Brown sugar contains 3 mcg. per gram of copper, while white refined sugar contains 0.08 mcg. per gram.

Nutritional surveys in the past have indicated that most diets

Copper Content of Selected Foods
Average adult requirement is 2–3 mg.

Food	Approximate Content (mg per 3 oz.)
Almonds	0.60
Applesauce	0.30
Avocado	0.35
Bacon	0.50
Banana	0.45
Barley	0.63
Beets	0.20
Brazil nuts	1.00
Bread, white	0.20
Bread, whole wheat	0.20
Brown sugar	0.27
Cashew nuts	0.70
Coconut	0.35
Corn	0.40
Chicken	0.25
Eggplant	0.27
Halibut	0.10
Hazelnuts	1.30
Honey	1.50
Kale	0.27
Lamb	0.22
Lentils	0.63
Calves liver	3.50
Lobster	2.00
Mushrooms	5.40
Mussels	2.90
Molasses, blackstrap	2.00
Oats	0.67
Oysters	3.10
Peanuts	0.65
Potatoes	0.13
Rice	0.35
Salmon	0.72
Seaweed	0.55

Copper Content of Selected Foods

Food	Approximate Content (mg per 3 oz.)
Shrimp	0.50
Spinach	0.80
Tuna	0.45
Turkey	0.16
Walnuts	0.80
Wheat germ	2.60

provide at least 2 mg. of copper per day. This, together with the amount that leaches into our water via copper pipes (which may be as much as 0.1–0.5 mg. per day) suggests that copper nutrition is adequate. Several recent surveys, however, have indicated that copper intakes with typical diets may be less than 1 mg. per day and the trend away from copper pipes is removing that source of copper. At present this controversy is unresolved, but since there are no overt signs of copper deficiencies, it would seem that our diets are providing a reasonable quantity of this mineral.

Deficiencies

Copper deficiencies are rare because the mineral is so widely distributed in our foods. However, iron, cadmium, and, surprisingly, vitamin C have been shown to decrease copper absorption. In addition, excessive doses of zinc can worsen an existing copper deficiency.

People with chronic diarrhea, malabsorption diseases, severe malnutrition, or kidney diseases, those receiving intravenous feedings for long periods of time without copper supplementation, and some patients who have had extensive bowel surgery may develop copper difficulties. Copper deficiencies have also been found in malnourished children who are fed milk diets (milk is not a particularly good source of copper).

Certain people are born with inherited copper deficiencies due to enzyme defects or impaired copper absorption mechanisms. One of these diseases is albinism, where the body is unable to make melanin, its natural skin coloring agent. The other is called Menke's kinky hair syndrome and is characterized by retarded growth, degeneration of the central nervous system, and sparse, brittle hair. Intravenous copper has been given to these children, but this has not been successful in prolonging their lives. Death usually occurs within a year after symptoms begin to develop.

Anemia is a major symptom of copper deficiency, and this is because copper is so necessary for iron to be absorbed, transported, and utilized. Deficiencies in animals result in impairment in bone formation, impairment in hair and wool formation, and disorders of the blood vessels and heart, especially degeneration and weakening of the aorta.·

In contrast to what we have seen with the other vitamins and minerals, oral contraceptive use seems to increase, rather than decrease, copper levels. Increased plasma copper levels are also noted during pregnancy and during acute and chronic infections and heart attacks. The significance of these observations to human health is unknown at present.

Hair analysis is sometimes used as a measure of copper nutrition because minerals are known to be stored in hair, but this is not a reliable test; urine or plasma copper levels must be used.

Toxicity

Copper toxicity can result from an intake of 10 mg. per day or more from any source, including foods or vitamin supplements. Symptoms of copper toxicity are nausea, vomiting, muscle aches, stomach pains, and, surprisingly, hemolytic anemia.

Wilson's disease, an inherited disorder, results in chronic copper toxicity. People with this disease slowly accumulate copper in their systems from birth because of a defect in the body's ability to remove copper via the liver. The condition causes progressive deterioration of mental function and loss of coordination. It also causes hemolytic anemia and liver damage and, if untreated, is fatal. Treatment involves restricted intake of copper-rich foods, the use of medicines to prevent the absorption of that copper which is ingested, and sometimes intravenous drugs to remove copper from the body.

Interactions

See the discussions under "Functions" and "Deficiencies."

Therapeutic Uses

There is no therapeutic use for copper supplements other than for relief of deficiency.

Unsubstantiated Claims

Heart Disease

One group of investigators believes that the zinc–copper ratio in our diets should be as low as possible to minimize the risk of heart diseases. A low ratio means roughly equivalent amounts of zinc and copper; a high ratio would mean more zinc than copper. This theory is based in part on the facts that (1) high-fiber diets, which are thought to lessen the risk of developing heart diseases, are high in phytic acid, which decreases the absorption of zinc; (2) exercise, which is known to decrease the risk of heart diseases, causes perspiration, which eliminates zinc; (3) copper deficiencies can increase cholesterol levels; and (4) zinc inhibits copper utilization.

The zinc–copper ratio theory is very speculative, but it does suggest caution for people who advocate routine zinc supplements for wound healing or other purposes. It is better to eat a varied diet to achieve adequate mineral nutrition than to take extra supplements that might upset the body's delicate mineral balance.

Arthritis

Copper bracelets have long been used for arthritis, but there is no good evidence that these have any benefit; the amount of copper absorbed would be very low. It is true, however, that copper is an important component of the enzyme superoxide dismutase, which may be protective against arthritis; recent investigations examined various organic copper complexes for possible antiarthritic activity.

Availability

Copper supplements are available in the form of 2.5 mg. tablets.

Fluoride

Fluoride is well known for its ability to help reduce tooth decay and cavities. Use of fluoride for this function is therapeutic; it is not done to correct nutritional fluoride deficiency. Supplementation of most municipal water supplies with fluoride has been carried out in the United States since the 1950s and is now common practice in many countries. This has conclusively decreased dental caries by 40 to 70 percent with no discernible harm.

Fluoride is available naturally as fluoride ion in soil and water supplies. It is presumed to be essential, although no deficiencies are known.

function

Fluoride is found mainly in teeth and bone, but its specific biochemical function is unknown. In teeth, it forms a tough outer layer, which makes it more difficult for bacteria to attack and cause tooth decay. In bones, it can replace calcium, but the quality of the bone is then not as good.

Daily Requirements

Nutritional requirements are unknown. Intakes range from 0.5–1.5 mg. in areas where the water contains no fluoride to 2–4 mg. per day in areas where the water supplies are fluoridated. Caries are prevented by daily intake of more than 1.5 mg. per day. Children who do not have access to fluoridated water or water with a naturally high fluoride content should be given supplements (tablets or liquid) to provide about 1 mg. per day. This is particularly important for very young children because fluoride supplements become less effective after the teeth have formed.

Dietary Sources

The fluoride content of foods varies tremendously. It is relatively high where soils are rich and local vegetables are consumed and where the drinking water (and cooking water) is fluoridated. Seafoods and fish products are often good sources, as is tea. Additional good sources are listed in the accompanying table, but the fluoride contents are only approximations because of the variability discussed above.

Fluoride Content of Selected Foods

Food	Approximate Content (mg. per 3 oz.)
Apples	0.80
Cod	0.70
Eggs	0.09
Kidneys	0.80
Calf's liver	0.13
Salmon	0.40
Sardines	1.00
Tea	0.30 per 8 oz. cup

Deficiencies

Under careful experimental conditions involving prolonged feeding of fluoride-deficient diets, deleterious effects were found in mice and rats, resulting in decreased growth and reproduction. No deficiencies are known in man.

Toxicity

Excess fluoride can cause problems. Adding more than two parts per million of fluoride to water supplies can lead to destruction of the teeth and to formation of fluoride deposits in the joints. However, most incidents of exposure to excess fluoride are usually caused by drinking water from deep wells that have been drilled through fluoride-containing rocks. These wells can contain fluoride far in excess of two parts per million. High fluoride doses, as could occur in poisoning, or fluoride overdose from taking too many sodium fluoride tablets can lead to convulsions and respiratory and cardiac failure.

Children who receive more than 20 mg. per day of fluoride over an extended period may develop fluoride toxicity (fluorosis). This results in discoloration, mottling, and weakening of the tooth enamel and permanent damage to the teeth.

Therapeutic Uses

The only proven use for fluoride is to prevent dental caries.

Unsubstantiated Claims

Some investigators have obtained benefit by giving fluoride supplements to patients with osteoporosis, while others have failed to show an improvement. More evaluation needs to be done.

Availability

Fluoride is available in tablets in strengths from 0.25 to 1 mg., drops in strengths from 0.125 to 0.25 mg. per drop, and as a topical rinse. Tablets and drops are best taken after meals and not together with milk or dairy products, which interfere with absorption. Fluoride rinses are sometimes used by dentists after cleaning of teeth.

Manganese

Manganese is an ''energy mineral'' that has also had some publicity as a possible deterrent to the aging process.

Function

Manganese is part of many body enzymes that are needed to generate energy; without manganese they could not function.

It is also a component of an enzyme called superoxide dismutase, which is involved in the regulation of oxygen level in body tissues. Excess oxygen can result in toxicity, which in turn results in destruction of body tissues. Superoxide dismutase prevents this by using up excess oxygen molecules.

Daily Requirements

There is no RDA value for manganese, although 2.5–5.0 mg. is considered to be a ''safe and adequate'' intake. The U.S. RDA value is 4 mg. ''Typical'' diets have been shown to provide 2–9 mg. on a daily basis.

Manganese Content of Selected Foods

Average adult requirement is 4 mg.

Food	Approximate Content (mg. per 3 oz.)
Almonds	1.70
Avocado	108.00
Bananas	0.60
Barley	3.00
Beets	0.55
Blackberries	0.60
Brazil nuts	2.80
Buckwheat	5.20
Chestnuts	3.40
Cloves	24.00
Coconut	1.20
Coffee beans	1.80
Flour, whole wheat	2.00
Ginger	8.00
Grapefruit	0.70
Green beans	0.30
Hazelnuts	3.80
Lettuce	0.70
Liver	0.30
Oatmeal	4.50
Parsley	0.85
Peanuts	1.30
Peas	1.80
Pecans	3.20
Rice	1.50
Seaweed	108.00
Spinach	0.75
Sunflower seeds	2.20
Tea	0.60
Watercress	1.80
Yams	0.45

Dietary Sources

Nuts, whole grains, seeds, fruits, and vegetables serve as excellent sources for manganese. Tea is surprisingly rich in manganese. Other good sources are listed in the accompanying table.

Deficiencies

Manganese deficiencies in animals result in depressed growth, skeletal abnormalities, decreased fertility, defects in carbohydrate and fat metabolism, abnormal gait, and an increase in clotting time for blood. Deficiencies in man are virtually unknown. There is only one reported case in which manganese deficiency was accidentally produced in a hospitalized patient who lost weight and developed low blood cholesterol, rash, and change in hair color.

Toxicity

Manganese toxicity has not been observed in people who eat foods rich in the mineral or in those who take it in supplemental form. However, psychiatric abnormalities and nerve disorders resembling Parkinson's disease have been seen in people exposed to manganese oxide dust at their jobs. Unfortunately, the nerve damage produced by manganese toxicity is permanent.

Therapeutic Uses

None.

Unsubstantiated Claims

Because of its role in controlling oxygen level and hence in halting destruction of body tissues, manganese, like selenium, has been promoted as an antiaging substance. Unfortunately, it is not.

Availability

Manganese is rarely used alone but is present in many vitamin-mineral combinations.

Molybdenum

Most people are familiar with gout, but many may not realize that little-known molybdenum plays a major role in cause and prevention of this painful ailment.

Function

Molybdenum is a component of xanthine oxidase, an enzyme involved in converting nucleic acid to uric acid, a waste product eliminated in the urine. Normal molybdenum level is necessary for this enzyme to handle its function properly. If there is too much molybdenum, and hence too much of this enzyme, too much uric acid can be produced. There is a limit to the amount of uric acid the kidneys can handle, and excess piles up in the blood. It is then deposited in the joints, where it crystallizes, causing the inflammatory condition called gout.

Molybdenum also functions on a see-saw basis with copper. If you have excess molybdenum, your copper level will drop; if you have excess copper, your molybdenum level will drop.

Daily Requirements

The molybdenum requirements in man are unknown but diets usually provide 90–350 mg. of molybdenum on a daily basis. A "safe and adequate" range is considered to be 150–500 mg. per day.

Dietary Sources

Accurate levels of molybdenum in common foods are not available. The composition of this element in foods is known to vary widely depending on the soil of origin. There are significant concentrations in meats, whole grains, and legumes.

Deficiencies

Molybdenum deficiencies in animals are very difficult to achieve even when special depleted diets are used. The only clear indication of deficiency is depressed activity of xanthine oxidase, but some animal studies have also shown an impairment in growth. Human deficiencies are unknown except for one reported case in a patient receiving long-term intravenous feeding. The symptoms were rapid heartbeat, rapid breathing, night blindness, and irritability.

Toxicity

Molybdenum is not considered toxic for most people, although Soviet researchers believe that excess amounts of molybdenum may cause a goutlike syndrome. One area in the Soviet Union where soils are very high in molybdenum (intakes in the 5,000–10,000 mg. per day range) has a high incidence of gout.

Interactions

For discussion of interaction with copper, see "Function."

Therapeutic Uses

Molybdenum has no proven therapeutic uses. Theoretically, a low molybdenum diet would depress xanthine oxidase, which would be of help in cutting down the excess uric acid produced by people with gout. This approach is probably impractical, however, because of the difficulty in obtaining a diet free of this trace mineral. Furthermore, a drug called allopurinol works well as an inhibitor of xanthine oxidase and is easy and safe to use.

Unsubstantiated Claims

None.

Availability

Supplements in the form of tablets and capsules are not generally available. Molybdenum is added to some multivitamin and mineral combinations but is not necessary. There is no reason to supplement with molybdenum.

Selenium

More and more research on selenium points out that it may be very important in human nutrition, not because deficiencies are common but because this mineral may aid in the prevention of some cancers.

Function

Selenium is a component of one form of an important enzyme called glutathione peroxidase. This enzyme sits in the fluid in and around body cells and inactivates substances called peroxides, which contain a high level of oxygen. Because excess oxygen can result in toxicity, which in turn can result in destruction of tissue, peroxides pose a threat to vital tissues and membranes. Left unchecked, they could destroy these tissues and cause cancer and even death.

Glutathione peroxidase is now thought to be our "first line of defense" against peroxidative damage. A second "line of defense" is vitamin E, which is located inside the membranes themselves. Thus, selenium and vitamin E go hand in hand in a protective role for the body.

Daily Requirements

Selenium requirements in man are not known with certainty. An estimated "safe and adequate" range is 50–200 mcg.

We are faced with a difficult situation when it comes to taking selenium supplements because the amounts needed are not known and most popular vitamin-mineral combinations do not contain selenium. Because of the toxicity you should keep your daily dose of selenium below 100 mcg. This, together with amounts found in your food, should be ample.

Dietary Sources

The selenium content of foods is highly variable because of the wide variability of this element in the soil, and accurate levels in foods are not available. Seafoods, organ meats, and whole grains are considered good sources, while fruits and vegetables are considered to be low in selenium. Refining of foods, cooking, and discarding of cooking water decrease selenium intake substantially.

Dietary surveys show an average intake of from 60 to 150 mcg. per day.

Deficiencies

Selenium deficiencies have been well studied in livestock and laboratory animals. Deficiencies in animals cause a variety of life-threatening conditions including infertility, muscular dystrophy, exudative diathesis in fowl, pancreatic fibrosis in chicks, hepatosis in pigs, and "unthriftiness" in sheep and cattle. These deficient states are much the same as those caused by deficiency of vitamin E, and large selenium doses will cure most, but not all, vitamin E deficiency symptoms. Since both vitamin E and selenium play a role in protecting against oxidative damage, it is not surprising that one can sometimes be substituted for the other.

Selenium deficiency in man is almost unknown, even in areas of the country where livestock are suffering from selenium deficiency. However, deficiency has been noted in a few patients with alcoholic cirrhosis and in a few patients receiving long-term intravenous nutrition without selenium; they suffered from heart problems that responded to selenium supplements. There is also speculation that Keshan's disease, a fatal heart disease seen in children living in certain sections of China, may be due to a selenium deficiency.

Toxicity

Selenium toxicity in animals can cause excess salivation, paralysis, blindness, and difficulty in breathing. Interestingly, human poisonings from foods grown in areas where livestock are being poisoned are not reported. Selenium poisonings have been discovered in several villages in China where droughts forced the villagers to eat high-selenium vegetables. Intakes were found to be 3,000–7,000 mcg. per day ("normal" is 50–150 mcg. per day). The villagers suffered hair and nail loss and problems of the nervous system.

Epidemiological studies have also shown a relationship between high levels of selenium in water and dental caries—the higher the selenium, the higher the caries rate.

Therapeutic Uses

Animal studies have conclusively demonstrated that selenium deficiencies increase the growth rate and numbers of tumors when cancer-causing chemicals are administered. High selenium intake seems to have a protective effect in these animal studies. Since the selenium-dependent enzyme glutathione peroxidase has a protective function against peroxidative damage, as discussed under "Function," it seems logical to assume that peroxidative damage must somehow lead to cancer.

In humans the only evidence that we have that selenium may protect against cancer is that obtained from broad-based epidemiological studies. If one compares the selenium content of the drinking water with death rates from cancer in various parts of the United States or even between countries, one finds the following relationship: the higher the selenium, the lower the rate of cancer. Obviously, other factors enter into this, and cancer in high-selenium areas is still a problem. It has been estimated that the risk for certain cancers is twice that in very low-selenium areas than that in high-selenium areas. High-selenium areas are to be found in parts of Wyoming, Alaska, Arkansas, Mississippi, South Dakota, and Colorado, while low-selenium areas are found in California, Ohio, Washington, Oregon, Pennsylvania, Indiana, and New York. Breast, colon, and lung cancers, our biggest killers, seem to be affected by selenium intake.

Zinc, cadmium, and copper counteract the effects of selenium in the body, and high intakes of these three minerals may inhibit the cancer-protecting effect of selenium, although there are no human studies to support this claim. Our advice is that it is better to take a mineral mixture balanced by Mother Nature in the form of whole grains and seafood than to fool around with potent mineral supplements—at least until more is known.

Because of the association of selenium deficiency and heart problems in humans, there is also interest in the therapeutic benefit of selenium supplements in heart disease. The answers are not yet in on this research.

Unsubstantiated Claims

Because of its role in controlling oxygen levels and hence halting destruction of body tissues, selenium, like manganese, has been erroneously promoted as an antiaging substance.

Availability

A few vitamin-mineral products contain selenium, and it is now becoming more available in tablet form as well.

12

Minor Trace Minerals

Very little is known about the role of the following trace elements in human nutrition, but research on animals has revealed a possible role for some of them.

Cadmium stimulates many enzyme systems, but none of them rely on cadmium alone; they are stimulated by other minerals as well. Cadmium toxicity has been reported in industrial workers who were exposed to cadmium dust. They developed a disease called Itai-Itai, which causes breathing difficulties.

Cobalt has been identified with a deficiency in humans. The deficiency symptoms are associated with its role as a component of Vitamin B_{12} (see p. 129). Cobalt toxicity can cause thyroid overgrowth in infants.

Nickel may interact with iron, but its exact function is unknown.

Silicon may play a role in the functioning of our connective tissue.

Vanadium is thought to play a role in the metabolism of our bones and teeth.

The functions of *tin* and *arsenic* in humans are not known.

13

Electrolytes

Sodium and Potassium

Sodium and potassium are not like other minerals, which are small amounts of inorganic material that act as catalysts for metabolic reactions in the body. Rather, sodium and potassium are considered "electrolytes," whose most important function is to maintain the proper amount of water inside and outside of cells.

Serious athletes who lose excessive amounts of sodium through perspiration and people with hypertension who lose excessive amounts of potassium through diuretics are most likely to be concerned about maintaining proper electrolyte balance.

Function

Sodium and potassium exist in and around cells as "ions" with a plus charge. In the water surrounding every cell the ratio of sodium to potassium is believed to be 31:1 inside every cell it is about 1:16. The usual "counter ion" with a negative charge is chloride (from chlorine).

Together, sodium and potassium provide the electrical potential that is necessary for cell membranes to exert their selectivity as to what they allow inside the cell and what they will exclude, including, of course, water. Nerve functions and muscle contractions also rely on the flow of sodium and potassium.

Daily Requirements

No RDA has been established for sodium or potassium, but it has been estimated that we need about 1,000 mg. of sodium a day (equivalent to 2,500 mg. of salt) and 2,000–6,000 mg. of potassium.

Dietary Sources

We all know of sources of salt in our diet—they are the highly processed foods many of us like so well, such as bacon, "instant" soups, bouillon, snack foods, canned goods, and ham. Additional high-sodium foods are listed in the accompanying table.

Sodium Content of Selected Foods

Food	Approximate Content (mg. per 3 oz.)
Apples, raw	0.9
Bacon	919.0
Bananas	0.9
Beef, dried	3,870.0
Beef, fresh ground	42.0
Bread, white	474.0
Bread, whole wheat	456.0
Butter	888.0
Cabbage	13.0
Clams	909.0
Green beans, canned	212.0
Green beans, cooked	4.0
Grapefruit	0.9
Ham	990.0
Margarine	888.0

Food	Approximate Content (mg. per 3 oz.)
Milk	45.0
Oranges	0.9
Potatoes	4.0
Raisins	24.0
Sardines	741.0
Squash	0.9
Tomatoes, canned	117.0
Tomatoes, fresh	3.0

Because of the American penchant for salty foods, a "typical" diet contains 3,000–7,000 mg., and "low-sodium" diets usually provide from 0.5 to 2,000 mg. of salt. Clearly, most of us would do well to decrease our sodium intake.

Because of the negative effect of excessive sodium on potassium balance, you need to consider both the potassium and sodium content of foods in your overall diet if you wish to increase or maintain body potassium levels. Most commercially canned vegetables have salt added to improve taste so that while they provide plenty of potassium, they also provide plenty of sodium and should be avoided. Clams, sardines, and lima beans are rich in potassium but also sodium. Good high-potassium, low-sodium sources are bananas, raisins, potatoes, tomatoes, apples, and oranges. Additional good sources are listed in the accompanying table.

Most diets provide 2–6 g. of potassium per day.

Potassium Content of Selected Foods

Food	Approximate Content (mg. per 3 oz.)
Apples, raw	99
Bacon	3
Bananas	333
Beef, dried	180
Beef, fresh, ground	405
Bread, white	246

Potassium Content of Selected Foods

Food	Approximate Content (mg. per 3 oz.)
Bread, whole wheat	95
Butter	21
Cabbage	93
Grapefruit	122
Green beans, canned	86
Green Beans, cooked	136
Margarine	21
Milk	130
Oranges	180
Peas, fresh, cooked	122
Potatoes	453
Raisins	687
Squash	127
Tomatoes	220

Deficiencies

Sodium deficiency is found mainly in situations of overexertion when perspiration losses of sodium are excessive but is also associated with many diseases. Generally, a strenuous workout on the first hot day is more likely to cause sodium depletion than continued exercise. Most people adapt to heat within a few days so that even though perspiration may continue, less sodium is lost. Symptoms of deficiency are muscle and stomach cramps, nausea, and fatigue. Sodium chloride tablets (one or two 1 g. tablets for the first few days) or a salt or electrolyte solution can be taken to prevent or relieve this.

Occasionally women on sodium-restricted diets during pregnancy can also develop the same problem as athletes or others involved in strenuous physical activity. Low salt diets help your body conserve calcium. If you need calcium supplementation, a low salt diet will make it more effective.

Potassium deficiencies usually occur for reasons other than a poor diet. Perhaps the most common reason for concern over potassium intake is the use of diuretic drugs that cause excessive loss of this element. However, this can be controlled to some extent by a low-sodium diet because the relationship between sodium and potassium in the kidneys determines the degree of excretion of each. Normally, large amounts of sodium are excreted with water while some potassium is retained. If there is little sodium to be excreted, much more potassium will be retained.

Another common cause of potassium deficiency is prolonged nausea or diarrhea; fluids in the gut are rich in potassium, and prolonged losses require potassium replacement. It is also possible to become deficient because of insufficient potassium in intravenous fluids, but this is unusual because most intravenous fluids are balanced in potassium and sodium content.

Symptoms of potassium deficiency include lethargy, a decrease in reflexes, muscle cramps and spasms, weakness, and most importantly, abnormal heartbeats that show up in the electrocardiogram. If a person already has heart disease, a potassium deficiency can make matters worse. Potassium deficiency can also cause increased sensitivity to the heart medications digoxin and digitoxin. Symptoms are the same as those for an overdose of digitoxin or digoxin, that is, nausea, vomiting, loss of appetite, abnormal heartbeats, and other symptoms of heart failure.

Toxicity

Most health authorities now agree that excessive salt intake increases the risk of high blood pressure. Of course, high blood pressure increases risk of heart disease, so, while salt certainly is not the only cause of heart disease, it is one factor that we can easily minimize. The rapidly disappearing practice of putting salt in baby foods sets up a pattern of increasing desire for salty foods which parents can combat at an early age by using low-salt foods for their children and discouraging the use of the salt shaker. If children did not acquire the taste or penchant for salted foods, minimizing salt intake during the adult years would not be such a problem.

Salt substitutes are formulated to replace the sodium ion in sodium chloride (salt) with some other ion, usually potassium. This works reasonably well, but the best procedure is to cut down on sodium intake.

An excess of potassium, resulting from an intake of over 18 g. a day, could occur through dietary intake, but this is unlikely; potassium toxicity is usually seen in patients taking potassium supplements incorrectly, or in cases of kidney failure. Symptoms are very much like those observed with a deficiency. Thus, muscle weakness, pain, abnormal heartbeats, and even heart failure may occur.

Calcium as calcium gluconate given intravenously or a special resin taken by mouth (Kayexolate) can be used to combat an excess of potassium.

Therapeutic Uses

Sodium or potassium supplements may be given to counteract any of the standard symptoms of deficiency reviewed earlier in this profile. However, such symptoms will not be alleviated by sodium or potassium unless they are, in fact, caused by electrolyte deficiency.

Unsubstantiated Claims

None.

Availability

Salt (sodium chloride) tablets of 1 g. each may be purchased without a prescription.

A large number of potassium products in both liquid and tablet form are available by prescription and should never be taken unless prescribed specifically for you. Use of some potassium tablets has caused local damage to the stomach and intestine, but such risk can be minimized by using a timed-release tablet or potassium solution.

Table 10
Mineral and Electrolyte Deficiency and Toxicity Symptoms

Mineral	Source	Deficiency	Toxicity
Cadmium	flour, rice, white sugar, coffee, tea	none known	breathing problems
Calcium	carob, cheese, milk, sardines, sesame seeds, some nuts, yogurt	osteomalacia, osteoporosis, rickets, seizures, muscle spasms	relatively non-toxic, but kidney stones may form in severe cases.

Electrolytes

Mineral	Source	Deficiency	Toxicity
Chromium	oysters, eggs, yeast, whole grains	very rare; disturbances in fat, sugar, and protein metabolism	relatively non-toxic in daily doses of 1,000 mg. or less. Industrial exposure can lead to lung cancer
Cobalt	(See vitamin B_{12}. Cobalt is a component of that vitamin.)		
Copper	shellfish, organ meat, fish, some vegetables	deficiency is rare; anemia, impaired bone and hair formation, retarded growth, and nervous system development.	nausea, vomiting, muscle aches, stomach pains, hemolytic anemia
Fluoride	seafood, liver, kidneys, tea	none known in humans	destruction of the teeth and bones
Iodine	seafood, milk, plants grown near the sea	childhood: slowed growth and sexual development, mental retardation, deafness, cretinism.	rash, headache, metallic taste, breathing difficulty, "iodide goiter"
Iron	liver, beef, egg yolks, nuts, seafood, whole grains	anemia, weakness, listlessness, pale skin coloration, swallowing difficulty, cracked lips or tongue, irritability	vomiting, cramps, diarrhea, weak pulse, exhaustion; severe overdoses can be deadly
Magnesium	molasses, nuts, fish, whole grains	convulsions, tremor, confusion, delirium, muscle spasms	toxicity is rare; diarrhea, fatigue, weakness, reduced heart and breathing rate

Mineral	Source	Deficiency	Toxicity
Manganese	nuts, whole grains, seeds, vegetables, fruits	very rare; skin rash, change in hair color	psychiatric and nerve disorders
Molybdenum	legumes, meats, whole grains	very rare; rapid breathing, night blindness, rapid heartbeat	nontoxic in humans
Nickel	vegetable oils	none known	none known
Phosphorous	Found in almost all foods. Fish, meats, and dairy products are good sources.	deficiency is rare; bone pain, loss of appetite, weakness, and brittle bones	toxicity is rare; brittle bones (due to calcium loss)
Potassium	canned vegetables, bananas, raisins, potatoes, tomatoes, apples, oranges	lethargy, weakness, poor reflexes, muscle cramps, spasms, abnormal heart rhythms	muscle weakness, pain, abnormal heart rhythms and possible failure. toxicity usually occurs after incorrect use of potassium supplement
Selenium	seafood, organ meats, whole grains	very rare; heart problems	tooth decay, nerve problems, hair and nail loss
Sodium	a wide variety of foods, but especially highly processed foods such as instant soups, snack foods, and canned goods	muscle and stomach cramps, nausea, fatigue	increased chance of high blood pressure, water retention, bloating
Vanadium	seafood	none known	none known
Zinc	meats, poultry, eggs, liver, seafood, whole grains	diarrhea, hair loss, slowed growth, loss of appetite, skin lesions, slowed sexual development	vomiting, stomach pain, tiredness, kidney failure, poor coordination

Part IV

VITAMIN, MINERAL, AND DRUG INTERACTIONS

The table on the following pages will provide you with information that, although known to physicians and pharmacists, has never been made generally available to the consumer. These tables will detail the possible effects that vitamins and minerals can have on each other, on the medicines you take, and on laboratory tests commonly prescribed by your doctor. For example, did you know any of the following facts?

• Women taking oral contraceptive pills (the pill) may have more vitamin A in their blood than nonusers and need more vitamin B_6 (pyridoxine).

• People taking digitalis drugs should avoid excess calcium, unless prescribed by their doctor, because the combination can lead to abnormal heart rhythms.

• People who take lithium to control manic depressive illness should avoid iodine supplements because they will experience an abnormal depression of thyroid gland function.

• People who take iron supplements should consider taking vitamin C with their iron because the vitamin will increase the amount of iron absorbed into the bloodstream.

• If you take an oral anticoagulant (blood-thinning) medicine, you should avoid megadoses of vitamin C because the vitamin can interfere with the effect of the anticoagulant by preventing it from passing from the stomach into the bloodstream.

• People who take isoniazid as a part of a treatment for tuberculosis or hydralazine for high blood pressure must take extra vitamin B_6.

If you take supplemental vitamins and/or are under any medical treatment, the following table contains essential information for you. Be sure also to inform your doctor of any vitamins you may be taking when you go for treatment.

Table 11

Vitamin, Mineral and Drug Interactions

	Can interact with:	to:
Vitamin B₁ **Thiamin**	drugs used to relax muscles during surgery	—produce excessive muscle relaxation. No special precautions are needed.
Vitamin B₂ **Riboflavin**	certain urine tests	—produce false elevations in urine tests for chemicals known as catecholamines. These chemicals are essential to nervous system function. —cause discoloration of the urine. Riboflavin can interfere with any test in which color is important because it gives the urine a yellowish discoloration.
Vitamin B₃ **Nicotinic Acid** (Niacin)	clonidine (Catapres) for hypertension	—eliminate flushing of the skin normally caused by nicotinic acid.
	certain blood tests	—elevate blood sugar. Very large doses of nicotinic acid must be taken to produce this effect. —increase growth hormone levels in the blood. —lower blood cholesterol (15–30 percent). Large daily doses of about 3 g. are required to give this effect. —increase blood uric acid levels. Large daily doses must be taken to produce this effect.

	Can interact with:	to:
		—increase blood levels of certain liver enzymes and chemicals. Nicotinic acid has been associated with jaundice in several patients.
	certain urine tests	—produce false elevations in urine tests for chemicals known as catecholamines. These chemicals are essential to nervous system function.
		—increase the amount of sugar in the urine. Large doses of nicotinic acid must be taken to produce this effect.
	barbiturate drugs	—increase the rate at which the barbiturate is broken down in the body.
	levodopa (l-dopa) for Parkinson's disease	—produce a dramatic interference in the effectiveness of levodopa. Doses as small as 10 mg. may produce this effect. Pyridoxine tablets or liquids and multivitamins containing pyridoxine should be avoided by people taking levodopa, unless carbidopa is also being taken, in which case the interaction does not occur.
Vitamin B$_6$ Pyridoxine	phenytoin (Dilantin) for seizures	—increase the rate at which the phenytoin is broken down in the body. Large doses of pyridoxine must be taken to produce this effect.
	isoniazid for tuberculosis	—produce pyridoxine deficiency. Extra pyridoxine is needed while taking this drug.

cycloserine for
tuberculosis

— produce pyridoxine deficiency. Conversely, pyridoxine may prevent nervous system side effects associated with cycloserine.

hydralazine (Apresoline)
for hypertension

— produce pyridoxine deficiency. Extra pyridoxine is needed while taking this drug.

penicillamine for arthritis
and Wilson's disease

— produce pyridoxine deficiency.

oral contraceptives

— produce pyridoxine deficiency. Extra pyridoxine is needed while taking oral contraceptives.

Vitamin B$_{12}$
Cyanocobolamine

vitamin B$_{12}$

— assist in the absorption of vitamin B$_{12}$.

aminosalicylic acid (PAS)
for tuberculosis

— prevent B$_{12}$ from passing from the gut into the bloodstream.

colcicine for gout

— lower amounts of B$_{12}$ passing from the gut into the blood.

chloramphenicol (Chloro-
mycetin), an antibiotic

— interfere with the effect of B$_{12}$ on the body.

neomycin, an antibiotic

— lower amounts of B$_{12}$ passing from the gut into the blood.

vitamin B$_6$

— assist in the absorption of vitamin B$_{12}$.

vitamin C

— assist in the absorption of vitamin B$_{12}$. If vitamin C is taken in normal doses. Large doses of vitamin C may destroy natural vitamin B$_{12}$ in food when mixed in the stomach.

	Can interact with:	to:
Folic Acid	chloramphenicol (Chloromycetin), an antibiotic	—produce folic acid deficiency
	pyrimethamine (Daraprim) for malaria	—interfere with the effectiveness of pyrimethamine. Patients taking pyrimethamine should *not* take extra folic acid.
	phenytoin for seizures	—decrease phenytoin effect. Patients taking phenytoin should avoid taking folic acid.
Vitamin C	"sulfa" drugs (antiinfective drugs)	—increase the chance of formation of drug crystals in the urine. Large doses of vitamin C are required to produce this effect.
	aminosalicylic acid (PAS) for tuberculosis	—increase the chance of formation of drug crystals in the urine. Large doses of vitamin C must be taken to produce this effect.
	antidepressant drugs	—decrease antidepressant effectiveness by making the body release the drug more quickly than normal.
	alcohol	—cause a slightly more rapid rate of breakdown of alcohol in the body. This could make you less sensitive to alcoholic beverages by removing alcohol from the blood more quickly. Large doses over a long period of time must be taken to produce this effect.

oral anticoagulant drugs, including warfarin	—interfere with anticoagulant effect. Very large doses (10 g. a day) of vitamin C could interfere with warfarin's passing from the gut into the bloodstream.
vitamin B_{12}	—assist in the absorption of vitamin B_{12}, if taken in normal doses. Large doses of vitamin C may destroy natural vitamin B_{12} in food when mixed in the stomach.
iron	—increase the amount of iron absorbed from non-meat foods.
calcium	—assist in the absorption of calcium.
copper	—decrease the absorption of copper. Large doses of vitamin C must be taken to produce this effect.
certain urine tests	—interfere with a test to determine the level of natural steroids in the urine. —give false reading on sugar in urine (either high or low). Large doses of vitamin C must be taken to produce this effect.
certain blood tests	—cause possible false reading of blood levels of bilirubin (one indication of liver function). —cause possible lower blood cholesterol readings in young persons (under age twenty-five) and higher readings in persons with a history of cholesterol problems.

	Can interact with:	to:
Vitamin A		—cause possible false reading indicating increase in level of uric acid. Large doses of vitamin C must be taken to produce this effect.
		—cause possible false negative test for blood in the stool.
	corticosteroid-type drugs (e.g. hydrocortisone, cortisone, prednisone, prednisolone betamethasone) for inflammation	—improve wound healing. Patients receiving corticosteroid drugs normally experience a slowness in wound healing. Topical vitamin A cream will reverse this effect, but vitamin A capsules or liquid taken orally will not.
	mineral oil	—interfere with vitamin A entering the blood. Do not take mineral oil within two hours of vitamin A.
	oral contraceptive pills	—produce higher than normal blood levels of vitamin A. The importance of this is not known.
	calcium	—assist in the absorption of calcium.
	vitamin E	—increase the capacity of body tissues to store vitamin A and therefore protect against vitamin A toxicity.
	certain blood tests	—produce high sedimentation rate (test for normal body reaction to injury or disease).
		—produce high prothrombin time (test for blood's ability to clot).

278

		—produce low white cell and red cell counts (tests for normal blood composition).
		—produce high levels of certain enzymes and chemicals found in the liver (general tests for liver function). Large doses of vitamin A must be taken to produce these effects.
	zinc	—assist in the absorption of vitamin A.
Vitamin D	phenytoin for seizures	—decrease vitamin D action in the body.
	barbiturates	—decrease vitamin D activity in the body. Long-term high doses of barbiturates must be taken to produce this effect.
	mineral oil	—interfere with vitamin D entering into the blood. Do not take mineral oil within two hours of vitamin D.
	certain blood tests	—interfere with the measurement of blood cholesterol levels.
		—increase blood levels of magnesium. This can be a severe problem in patients with kidney disease, in whom magnesium can be toxic.
Vitamin E	oral anticoagulant drugs	—produce bleeding. Large doses of vitamin E have been reported to interfere with the clotting mechanism, and therefore they enhance the effect of anticoagulants.
	iron	—interfere, possibly, with the effectiveness of iron therapy in anemic persons. This effect has been reported in children.
	vitamin A	—increase capacity of body tissues to store vitamin A and thereby protect against vitamin A toxicity.

	Can interact with:	to:
Vitamin K	oral anticoagulant drugs	—decrease anticoagulant action. This is a well-known effect. In fact, vitamin K is used as an antidote in overdosage of oral anticoagulants.
Calcium	digitalis drugs for heart failure	—produce abnormal heart rhythms. Large doses of calcium are needed to produce this effect. Patients taking a digitalis drug should not take supplementary calcium in large amounts.
	tetracycline, an antibiotic	—decrease the amount of tetracycline being absorbed into the blood. Do not take calcium and tetracycline within two hours of each other and avoid combining them with milk or other dairy products.
	vitamin C	—assist in the absorption of calcium.
	phosphorous	—maintain the appropriate ratio of calcium and phosphorous in the body.
	certain blood tests	—produce high serum amylase (test used to evaluate the pancreas). This effect requires consistently high blood levels of calcium. —interfere with test for blood levels of magnesium or actually lower blood levels of magnesium in some people.
	certain urine tests	—interfere with test for levels of naturally occurring steroids in the urine.

Phosphorous	calcium	—maintain appropriate ratio of phosphorous to calcium in the body.
Magnesium	drugs used to relax muscles during surgery	—produce excessive muscle relaxation. This interaction can produce serious difficulties. Although it has only been reported with intravenous magnesium preparations, people taking routine magnesium supplements should report this fact to their doctor prior to surgery.
	oral anticoagulant drugs	—lower anticoagulant effect. Magnesium may interfere with the passage of the anticoagulant into the blood from the gut.
	chlorpromazine (Thorazine), a tranquilizer	—lower chlorpromazine effectiveness. Magnesium may interfere with the passage of chlorpromazine into the blood from the gut.
Iron	allopurinol (Zyloprim) for gout	—increase iron storage in the liver. Do not take this combination.
	antacids	—decrease the amount of iron absorbed into the blood from the gut. Those two should be ingested at least two hours apart.
	chloramphenicol (chloromycetin), an antibiotic	—interfere with iron effectiveness in anemic people.
	cholestyramine resin (Questran) for cholesterol	—decrease the amount of iron absorbed into the blood from the gut. Do not take iron and cholestyramine within two hours of each other.

Can interact with:	to:
pancreatic extract (Pancreatin) for enzyme replacement	—decrease the amount of iron absorbed from the gut.
penicillamine (Cuprimine, Depen) for rheumatoid arthritis	—decrease the amount of penicillamine absorbed into the blood.
tetracycline	—interfere with the amount of tetracycline absorbed into the blood. Take these two at least two hours apart.
vitamin C	—increase the amount of iron absorbed into the bloodstream. Large doses of vitamin C must be taken to produce this effect.
vitamin E	—interfere with the effectiveness of iron therapy in anemic persons. This effect has been reported in children.
calcium	—assist in the absorption of calcium.
copper	—decrease the absorption of copper.
zinc	—decrease the absorption of iron. Large doses of zinc must be taken to produce this effect.

282

Iodine lithium carbonate for manic depressive illness

—produce abnormally low thyroid activity. Lithium patients should avoid iodine, which will suppress the thyroid gland.

certain blood tests

—interfere with tests for thyroid function.

certain urine tests

—interfere with test for levels of naturally occurring steroids in the urine.
—interfere with tests for thyroid function, if it is taken for other purposes.

Zinc tetracycline

—decrease the amount of tetracycline being absorbed into the bloodstream. Zinc and tetracycline should not be mixed; take these two at least two hours apart

vitamin A

—assist in the absorption of vitamin A.

copper

—decrease the absorption of copper. Large doses of zinc must be taken to produce this effect.

iron

—decrease the absorption of iron. Large doses of zinc must be taken to produce this effect.

vitamin C

—decrease the absorption of copper. Large doses of vitamin C must be taken to produce this effect.

Copper

molybdenum

—maintain the appropriate ratio of copper to molybdenum in the body.

	Can interact with:	to:
	iron	—decrease the absorption of copper.
	zinc	—decrease the absorption of copper. Large doses of zinc must be taken to produce this effect.
Molybdenum	copper	—maintain the appropriate ratio of molybdenum and copper in the body.

Bibliography

Adams, P. W., et al. Effect of pyridoxine hydrochloride (vitamin B_6) upon depression associated with oral contraceptives. *Lancet* (1973) 1:889–904.

Adams, P. W., et al. Vitamin B_6, depression and oral contraception. *Lancet* (1974) 2:516–17.

Ahmad, F., and Bamji, M. S. Vitamin supplements to women using oral contraceptives. *Contraception* (1976) 14:309–318.

Alhadeff, L., Gualtieri, C. T., and Lipton, M. Toxic effects of water soluble vitamins. *Nutrition Review* (1984) 42:33–40.

Anderson, B. B., et al. Effect of riboflavin on red-cell metabolism of vitamin B_6. *Nature* (1976) 253:574–575.

Anderson, B. M., Gibson, R. S., and Sabry, J. H. The iron and zinc status of long-term vegetarian women. *American Journal of Clinical Nutrition* (1981) 34:1042–1048.

Anderson, T. W., Reid, D.B.S., and Beatson, G. H. Vitamin C and the common cold: A double blind trial. *Canadian Medical Association Journal* (1972) 107:503.

Anderson, T. W., and Reid, P. B. A double blind trial of vitamin E in angina pectoris. *American Journal of Clinical Nutrition* (1974) 27:1174–1177.

285

Anderson, T. W., Surany, G., and Beatson, G. H. The effect on winter illness of large doses of vitamin C. *Canadian Medical Association Journal* (1974) 111:31.

Anon. Alcohol and the enterohepatic circulation of folate. *Nutrition Review* (1980) 38:220–223.

Anon. Calcium for post-menopausal osteoporosis. *Medical Letter on Drugs and Therapeutics* (1982) 24:105–106.

Anon. *Caloric and Selected Nutrient Values for Persons 1–74 Years of Age*. U.S. Department of Health and Welfare Publication No. (PHS) 79-1658. Hyatsville, Md.: National Center for Health Statistics, 1979.

Anon. Megavitamin E supplementation and vitamin K dependent carboxylation. *Nutrition Review* (1983) 41:268–270.

Anon. Niacin intoxication from pumpernickel bagels. New York: *Morbidity & Mortality Weekly Reports* (June 17, 1983) 32:305.

Anon. *Nutritive Value of American Foods*. Washington, D.C.: U.S. Department of Agriculture, 1975.

Anon. *Recommended Dietary Allowances*. 9th ed. Washington, D.C.: National Academy of Sciences, 1980.

Anon. Vegetarian diet and vitamin B_{12} deficiency. *Nutrition Review* (1978) 36:243–244.

Anon. Vitamin K, vitamin E and the coumarin drugs. *Nutrition Review* (1982) 40:180–182.

Ansell, J. E., Kumar, R., and Deykin, D. The spectrum of vitamin K deficiency. *Journal of the American Medical Association* (1977) 238:40–42.

Arlette, J. P. Zinc and the skin. *Pediatric Clinics of North America* (1983) 30:583–596.

Ascione, F. (Project Director). *Evaluations of Drug Interactions*. 2nd ed. Washington, D.C.: American Pharmaceutical Association, 1976.

Avioli, L. V. Effects of chronic corticosteroid therapy on mineral metabolism and calcium absorption. *Advances in Experimental Medicine & Biology* (1984) 171:381–397.

Avioli, L. V., and Haddad, J. G. The vitamin D family revisited. *New England Journal of Medicine* (1984) 311:47–49.

Ayers, S., and Mikan, R. Nocturnal leg cramps (systremma): A progress report on response to vitamin E. *Southern Medical Journal* (1974) 67:1308–1312.

Bibliography

Ayers, S., et al. Vitamin E as a useful therapeutic agent. *Journal of the American Academy of Dermatology* (1982) 7:521–525.

Ban, T. A., and Lehmann, H. E. Nicotinic acid in the treatment of schizophrenia. *Canadian Psychology Association Journal* (1975) 20:193–212.

Bankier, A., et al. Pyridoxine dependent seizures: A wider clinical spectrum. *American Journal of Disabled Children* (1983) 58:415–418.

Barkin, J. S., et al. Potassium chloride and gastrointestinal injury (letter). *Annals of Internal Medicine* (1983) 98:261–262.

Bender, J. F., Grove, W. R., and Fortner, C. L. High dose methotrexate with folinic acid rescue. *American Journal of Hospital Pharmacy* (1977) 34:961–965.

Bergen, J. C., and Bron, P. T. Nutritional status of "new" vegetarians. *Journal of the American Dietetic Association* (1980) 76:151–155.

Bickle, D. D. Calcium absorption and vitamin D metabolism. *Clinical Gastroenterology* (1983) 12:380–394.

Bierei, J. G. The role of vitamin E in clinical medicine. *ASDC J. Dent. Child.* (1984) 51:133–136.

Binder, H., et al. Tocopherol deficiency in man. *New England Journal of Medicine* (1965) 283:1289–1297.

Bjelke, E. Dietary vitamin A and human lung cancer. *International Journal of Cancer* (1975) 15:561–565.

Baird, I. M., et al. The effects of ascorbic acid and flavinoids on the occurrence of symptoms normally associated with the common cold. *American Journal of Clinical Nutrition* (1979) 32:1686–1690.

Blass, J. P., and Gilson, G. F. Abnormality of a thiamin requiring enzyme in patients with Wernicke-Korsakoff syndrome. *New England Journal of Medicine* (1977) 297:1367–1370.

Bollag, W. Vitamin A and retinoids: From nutrition to pharmacotherapy in dermatology and oncology. *Lancet* (1983) 1:860–863.

Bosse, T. R., and Donald, E. A. The vitamin B_6 requirement in oral contraceptive users: I. Assessment by pyridoxal level and transferase activity in erythrocytes. *American Journal of Clinical Nutrition* (1979) 32:1015–1023.

Bound, J. P. Spina bifida and vitamins (letter). *British Medical Journal* (1983) 286:147.

Bowerman, S. J., et al. Nutrient consumption of individuals taking or not taking nutrient supplements. *Journal of the American Dietetic Association* (1983) 82:401–404.

Boxer, L. A., et al. Projection of granulocytes by vitamin E in glutathine synthetase deficiency. *New England Journal of Medicine* (1979) 301:901–905.

Brace, L. The pharmacology and therapeutics of vitamin K. *American Journal of Medical Technology* (1983) 49:457–463.

Breslau, N. A., et al. Hypercalcemia associates with increased serum calcitriol levels in three patients with lymphoma. *Annals of Internal Medicine* (1984) 100:1–7.

Brewer, G. J., et al. Biological roles of ionic zinc. *Progress in Clinical Biological Research* (1983) 129:35–51.

Brewer, G. J., et al. Oral zinc therapy for Wilson's disease. *Annals of Internal Medicine* (1983) 99:314–319.

Brickman, A. S., et al. 1,25-dyhydroxy-vitamin D_3 in normal man and patients with renal failure. *Annals of Internal Medicine* (1974) 80:161–168.

Bright, S. E. Vitamin C and cancer prevention. *Seminars in Oncology* (1983) 10:294–298.

Brin, M., and Bauerin, F. Vitamin needs of the elderly. *Postgraduate Medicine* (1978) 63:155–163.

Brooke, O. G. Supplementary vitamin D in infancy and childhood. *Archives of Diseases in Children* (1983) 58:573–574.

Brookes, G. B. Vitamin D deficiency—a new cause of cochlear deafness. *Journal of Laryngology and Otolaryngology* (1983) 97:405–420.

Brown, E. D., Chan, W., and Smith, J. C. Bone demineralization during a developing zinc deficiency. *Proceedings of the Royal Society of Experimental Biology and Medicine* (1978) 157:211–214.

Bruns, M. E., and Bruns, D. E. Vitamin D metabolism and function during pregnancy. *Annals of Clinical Laboratory Science* (1983) 13:521–530.

Cameron, E., and Pauling, L. Supplemental ascorbate in the support and treatment: Prolongation of survival times in terminal cancer. *Proceedings of the National Academy of Science USA* (1978) 25:4538–4542.

Bibliography

Carney, M. W., et al. Thiamin, riboflavin and pyridoxine deficiency in psychiatric in-patients. *British Journal of Psychology* (1982) 141:271–272.

Carpenter, T. O., Carnes, D. L., and Anast, C. A. Hypoparathyroidism in Wilson's disease. *New England Journal of Medicine* (1983) 309:873–877.

Centerwall, B. S., and Criqui, M. H. Prevention of Wernicke-Korsakoff syndrome: A cost-benefit analysis. *New England Journal of Medicine* (1978) 299:285–289.

Cheraskin, E., Ringsdorf, W. M., and Sisley, E. *The Vitamin C Connection*. New York: Harper & Row, 1983.

Chien, L. T., et al. Harmful effect of megadoses of vitamins: Electroencephalogram abnormalities and seizures induced by folate in drug treated epileptics. *American Journal of Clinical Nutrition* (1975) 28:51–58.

Cholst, I. N., et al. The influence of hypermagnesemia on serum calcium and parathyroid hormone levels in human subjects. *New England Journal of Medicine* (1984) 310:1221–1225.

Chow, C. K., Dietary vitamin E and cellular susceptibility to cigarette smoking. *Annals of the New York Academy of Science* (1982) 393:96–108.

Coburn, S. P., et al. Effect of megavitamin treatment on mental performance and plasma vitamin B_6 concentrations in mentally retarded young adults. *American Journal of Clinical Nutrition* (1983) 18:353–355.

Cochrane, W. A., Overnutrition in prenatal and neonatal life: A problem? *Journal of the American Medical Association* (1965) 93:893–899.

Corash, L., et al. Reduced chronic hemolysis during high dose vitamin E administration in glutathione synthetase deficiency. *New England Journal of Medicine* (1980) 303:416–420.

Corrigan, J. J., and Marcus, F. I. Coagulopathy associated with vitamin E ingestion. *Journal of the American Medical Association* (1974) 230:1300–1301.

Coulehan, J. L., et al. Vitamin C and acute illness in Navajo school children. *New England Journal of Medicine* (1976) 295:973.

Coulehan, J. S., et al. Vitamin C prophylaxis in a boarding school. *New England Journal of Medicine* (1974) 290:6.

Creagan, E. T., et al. Failure of high dose vitamin C (ascorbic acid) therapy to benefit patients with advanced cancer: A controlled trial. *New England Journal of Medicine* (1979) 30:687–690.

Cromwell, G. F., et al. Pyridoxine dependent seizures. *American Family Physician* (1983) 27:183–187.

Cummings, F. J., et al. Changes in plasma vitamin A in lactating and non-lactating oral contraceptive users. *British Journal of Obstetrics and Gynaecology* (1983), 90:73–77.

Dannenberg, J. L. Vitamin C enamel loss (letter). *Journal of the American Dental Association* (1982) 105:172.

Darby, W. J., McNutt, J. W., and Todhunter, E.W. Niacin. *Nutrition Review* (1975) 33:289–297.

DeCosse, J. J. Effect of ascorbic acid on rectal polyps of patients with familial polyposis. *Surgery* (1975) 78:608–612.

DeCosse, J. J., Condon, R. E., and Adams, M. B. Surgical and medical measures in the prevention of large bowel cancer. *Cancer* (1977) 40:2549–2552.

Diem, K., and Lentner, C., eds. *Scientific Tables*. Ardsley, N.Y.: Geigy Pharmaceuticals, 1970.

Dietz, R. The role of potassium in hypertension. Discovery of potassium as a natriuretic and hypertensive agent. *American Journal of Nephrology* (1983) 3:100–108.

DiPalma, J. R., and Ritchie, D. M. Vitamin toxicity. *Annual Review of Pharmacology and Toxicology* (1977) 17:133–148.

Donald, E. A., and Bosse, T. R. The vitamin B_6 requirement in oral contraceptive users: II. Assessment by tryptophan metabolites, vitamin B_6 and pyridoxic acid levels in urine. *American Journal of Clinical Nutrition* (1979) 32: 1024–1032.

Dong, A., et al. Serum vitamin B_{12} and blood cell values in vegetarians. *Annals of Nutrition and Metabolism* (1982) 25:209–216.

Driscoll, R. H., et al. Vitamin D deficiency and bone disease in patients with Crohn's disease. *Gastroenterology* (1983) 28:145–53.

Dustan, H. P. Is potassium deficiency a factor in the pathogenesis and maintenance of hypertension? *Arteriosclerosis* (1983) 3:307–309.

Dutta, S. K., et al. Deficiency of fat-soluble vitamins in treated patients with pancreatic insufficiency. *Annals of Internal Medicine* (1982) 97:549–552.

Dworken, H. J. Vitamin E reconsidered. *Annals of Internal Medicine* (1983) 98:253–254.

Dychner, T., et al. Effect of magnesium on blood pressure. *British Medical Journal* (1983) 286:1847–1849.

Ebon, M. *The Essential Vitamin Counter*. New York: Bantam Books, 1979.

Ellis, J. M., et al. Response of vitamin B_6 deficiency and the carpal tunnel syndrome to pyridoxine. *Proceedings of the National Academy of Science USA* (1982) 79:7494–7498.

Ellis, J. M., et al. Survey and new data on treatment with pyridoxine of patients having a clinical syndrome including carpal tunnel and other defects. *Research Communications in Chemistry, Pathology and Pharmacology* (1977) 17:165–177.

Elwood, P. C., et al. A randomized controlled trial of the therapeutic effect of vitamin C in the common cold. *Practitioner* (1977) 218:133.

Elwood, P. C., et al. A randomized controlled trial of vitamin C in the prevention and amelioration of the common cold. *British Journal of Preventive and Social Medicine* (1976) 30:193.

Evans, D. L., et al. Organic psychosis without anemia or spinal cord symptoms in patients with vitamin B_{12} deficiency. *American Journal of Psychiatry* (1983) 140:218–221.

Farrel, P. M., and Bieri, J. G. Megavitamin E supplementation in man. *American Journal of Clinical Nutrition* (1975) 28:1381–1386.

Feldman, S., et al. Antacid effects on the gastrointestinal absorption of riboflavin. Publication in pp. (1983) 72:121–123.

Finn, N. N., et al. Effect of intramuscular vitamin E on frequency and severity of retrolental fibroplasia. *Lancet* (1982) 1:1087–1091.

Fisher, Michelle, and Lachance, Paul. Nutritional evaluation of published weight-reducing diets. *Journal of the American Medical Association* (1984) 85:450–454.

Fletcher, D. C. Vitamin K content of various foods. *Journal of the American Medical Association* (1977) 237:1871.

Foulkes, M. D. An antilactogenic effect of pyridoxine. *Journal of Obstetrics and Gynaecology of the British Commonwealth* (1973) 80:718–720.

Frannson, G. B., et al. Zinc, copper, calcium and magnesium in human milk. *Journal of Pediatrics* (1982) 10:504–508.

Fregly, M. J. Estimates of sodium and potassium intake. *Annals of Internal Medicine* (1983) 98:792–799.

Fumrich, R. M., et al. Hypervitaminosis A. A case report in an adolescent soccer player. *American Journal of Sports Medicine* (1983) 11:24–27.

Garry, P. J., et al. Nutritional status in a healthy elderly population: Riboflavin. *American Journal of Clinical Nutrition* (1982) 36:902–909.

Gaut, Z. N. Vitamin D metabolism and metabolic bone disease. *Current Concepts in Nutrition* (1983) 12:29–47.

Gillilan, R. E., and Modell, B. Quantitative evaluation of vitamin E in the treatment of angina pectoris. *American Heart Journal* (1977) 93:444–449.

Glusman, M. The syndrome of "burning feet" (nutritional metalgia) as a manifestation of nutritional deficiency. *American Journal of Medicine* (1947) 3:211–216.

Goodhart, R. S., and Shils, M. E., eds. *Modern Nutrition in Health and Disease.* Philadelphia: Lee and Febiger, 1980.

Goodman, D. S. Vitamin A and retinoids in health and disease. *New England Journal of Medicine* (1984) 310:1023–1031.

Goodman, D. S. Vitamin A metabolism. *Federation Proceedings* (1980) 39:2716–2722.

Gossell, T. A., and Wuest, J. R. Vitamins and minerals. *U.S. Pharmacist* (1982) 7:8–11.

Graham, S. Toward a dietary prevention of cancer. *Epidemiology Review* (1983) 5:38–50.

Gram, L. F., et al. Imipramine metabolism: pH dependent distribution and urinary excretion. *Clinical Pharmacology and Therapeutics* (1971) 12:239.

Gray, G. E., et al. Dietary intake and nutrient supplement use in a Southern California retirement community. *American Journal of Clinical Nutrition* (1983) 38:122–128.

Greengard, P. "The water soluble vitamins." In *The Pharmacological Basis of Therapeutics,* L. S. Goodman, ed. and A. Gillamn. 6th ed. New York: Macmillan, 1980.

Bibliography

Greentree, L. B. Dangers of vitamin B_6 in nursing mothers. *New England Journal of Medicine* (1979) 300:141–142.

Griffith, L. D., et al. Increasing prothrombin times in a warfarin treated patient upon withdrawal of Ensure Plus (letter). *Critical Care Medicine* (1982) 10:799–800.

Griffiths, L. L., and Scott, D. L. A double blind study for the detection of vitamin deficiencies in elderly patients in the hospital. *Vitamins 2* (Roche Laboratories, Nutley, N.J.) (1970).

Grubbs, C. J., et al. Inhibition of mammary cancer by retinyl methyl ether. *Cancer Research* (1977) 37:599–602.

Haeger, K. Long-time treatment of intermittent claudication with vitamin E. *American Journal of Clinical Nutrition* (1974) 27:1179–1181.

Haeger, K. The treatment of peripheral occlusive arterial disease with tocopherol as compared with vasodilator agents and antiprothrombin (dicumarol). *Vascular Diseases* (1968) 5:199–213.

Hallberg, L. Iron requirements and availability of dietary iron. *Experientia* (1983) 44:223–244.

Hambridge, K. M., et al. Zinc nutritional status during pregnancy. A longitudinal study. *American Journal of Clinical Nutrition* (1983) 37:429–442.

Hansten, P. D. *Drug Interactions.* 7th ed. Philadelphia: Lea and Febiger, 1979.

Harding, A. E., et al. Spinocerebellar degeneration secondary to chronic intestinal malabsorption: a vitamin E deficiency. *Annals of Neurology* (1972) 12:419–423.

Haussler, M. R., and McCain, T. A. Basic and clinical concepts related to vitamin D metabolism and action. *New England Journal of Medicine* (1980) 297:1041–1050.

Heaney, R. P., et al. Calcium nutrition and bone health in the elderly. *American Journal of Clinical Nutrition* (1982) 36:986–1013.

Henzel, J. H., DeWeese, M. S. and Lichiti, E. L. Zinc concentrations within healing wounds. *Archives of Surgery* (1970) 100:349–357.

Heidbreder, G., and Christophers, E. Therapy of psoriasis with retinoid plus PUVA: Clinical and histologic data. *Archives of Dermatology Research* (1979) 264:331–337.

Hem, S. L., et al. Evaluation of antacid suspensions containing aluminum hydroxide and magnesium hydroxide. *American Journal of Hospital Pharmacy* (1982) 39:1925–1930.

Herbert, V. Pangamic acid (vitamin B_{15}). *American Journal of Clinical Nutrition* (1979) 32:1534–1540.

Herbert, V., Gordon, A., and Coleman, N. Mutagenicity of dichloracetate, an ingredient in some formulations of pangamic acid (tradenamed "vitamin B_{15}"). *American Journal of Clinical Nutrition* (1980) 33:1179–1182.

Herbert, V., and Jacob, E. Destruction of vitamin B_{12} by ascorbic acid. *Journal of the American Medical Association* (1974) 230:241–242.

Hermann, W. J. The effect of vitamin E on lipoprotein cholesterol distribution. *Annals of the New York Academy of Science* (1982) 393:467–472.

Herold, E., Mattin, J. and Sabry, Z. Effect of vitamin E on human sexual functioning. *Sexual Behavior* (1979) 8:397–403.

Herzlich, B., and Herbert, V. The role of the pancreas in cobolamin (vitamin B_{12}) absorption. *American Journal of Gastroenterology* (1984) 79:489–493.

Heyden, S., et al. The role of potassium manipulation in blood pressure control. *Arteriosclerosis* (1983) 3:302–306.

Higginbottom, M. C., Sweetman, L., and Nuhan, W. L. A syndrome of methylmalonic acidurea and neurologic abnormalities of a vitamin B_{12} deficient breast-fed infant of a strict vegetarian. *New England Journal of Medicine* (1978) 299:317–323.

Hines, J. D. Megaloblastic anemia in an adult vegan. *American Journal of Clinical Nutrition* (1966) 19:260–268.

Hittner, H. M., et al. Retrolental fibroplasia: efficacy of vitamin E in a double blind study of preterm infants. *New England Journal of Medicine* (1981) 305:1365–1371.

Hodges, R. E. Vitamin C and cancer. *Nutrition Review* (1982) 40:289–292.

Hodges, R. E., et al. Human pantothenic acid deficiency produced by omega-methyl pantothenic acid. *Journal of Clinical Investigation* (1959) 38:1421–1425.

Hoffer, A. Megavitamin B therapy for schizophrenia. *Canadian Psychology Association Journal* (1971) 16:499–504.

Hoffman, K. J., Milne, F. J. and Schmidt, C. Acne hypervitamins and hypercalcemia. *South African Medical Journal* (1978) 54:579–580.

Hoffstrand, A. V. Pathology of folate deficiency. *Proceedings of the Royal Society of Medicine* (1977) 70:82–84.

Holmes, R. P., et al. The relationship of adequate intake of vitamin D to health and disease. *Journal of the American College of Nutrition* (1983) 2:173–199.

Horwitt, M. K. Therapeutic uses of vitamin E in medicine. *Nutrition Review* (1980) 38:105–113.

Horwitt, M. K. Vitamin E: A re-examination. *American Journal of Clinical Nutrition* (1976) 29:569–577.

Hotz, W. Nicotinic acid and its derivatives: A short survey. *Advances in Lipid Research* (1983) 20:195–217.

Hoyumpa, A. M., et al. Thiamin transport across the rat intestine. I: Normal characteristics. *Gastroenterology* (1975) 68:1217–1227.

Hoyumpa, A. M., et al. Thiamin transport across the rat intestine. II: Effects of ethanol. *Journal of Laboratory and Clinical Medicine* (1975) 86:803–813.

Hutton, C. W., et al. Assessment of the zinc-nutritional status of selected elderly subjects. *Journal of the American Dietetic Association* (1983) 82:148–153.

Iseri, L. T., and French, J. H. Magnesium: Nature's physiologic calcium blocker. *American Heart Journal* (1984) 108:188–193.

Ivy, M., and Elmer, G. Nutritional supplements, mineral and vitamin products. In *Handbook of Non-Prescription Drugs*. Washington, D.C.: American Pharmaceutical Association, 1982.

Jameson, S. Zinc nutrition and human pregnancy. *Progress in Clinical Biological Research* (1983) 129:35–51.

Jansen, J. D. Nutrition and cancer. *World Review of Nutrition and Diet* (1982) 39:1–22.

Jett, S. F. Vitamins in the prevention of neoplasms. *American Pharmacy* (1983) n.s.23:21–26.

Karlowski, T. R., et al. Ascorbic acid for the common cold. *Journal of the American Medical Association* (1975) 231:1038.

Kasa, R. M. Vitamin C: From scurvy to the common cold. *American Journal of Medical Technology* (1983) 49:23–26.

Keith, R. E., et al. Lung function and treadmill performance of smoking and nonsmoking males receiving ascorbic acid supplements. *American Journal of Clinical Nutrition* (1982) 36:840–845.

Klevay, L. M. Coronary heart disease: The zinc/copper hypothesis. *American Journal of Clinical Nutrition* (1975) 28:764–774.

Klevay, L. M., et al. The human requirement for copper. I: Healthy men fed a conventional American diet. *American Journal of Clinical Nutrition* (1980) 33:45–50.

Knudson, A. G., and Rothman, P. E. Hypervitaminosis A. *American Journal of Diseases of Children* (1953) 85:316–334.

Krawitt, E. L. Ethanol inhibits intestinal calcium transport in rats. *Nature* (1973) 243:13.

Krebs, H. A., Hems, R., and Tyler, B. The regulation of folate and methionine metabolism. *Biochemistry Journal* (1976) 158:341–353.

Kummet, T., and Meyskens, F. L. Vitamin A: A potential inhibitor of human cancer. *Seminars in Oncology* (1983) 10:281–289.

Kummet, T., Moon, T. E., and Meyskens, F. L. Vitamin A: Evidence for its preventive role in human cancer. *Nutrition and Cancer* (1983) 5:96–106.

Kwee, I. L., and Nakada, T. Wernicke's encepalopathy induced by tolazamide. *New England Journal of Medicine* (1983) 309:599–600.

Lande, N. I. More on the dangers of vitamin B_6 in nursing mothers. *New England Journal of Medicine* (1979) 300:926–927.

Langford, H. G. Dietary potassium and hypertension: Epidemiologic data. *Annals of Internal Medicine* (1983) 98:770–772.

Lee, C. J., Fowler, G. S., and Johnson, G.G.H. Effects of supplementation of the diet with calcium and calcium-rich foods on bone density in elderly females with osteoporosis. *American Journal of Clinical Nutrition* (1981) 34:819–823.

Lee, W. H. For many health beneficial reasons: Think zinc! *American Druggist* (1984) 189:64.

Legha, S. S., et al. Clinical and pharmacologic investigation of the effects of alpha-tocopherol on adriamycin cardiotoxicity. *Annals of the New York Academy of Science* (1982) 393:411–418.

Bibliography

Lehr, K., et al. Total body potassium depletion and the need for preoperative nutritional support in Crohn's disease. *Annals of Surgery* (1982) 196:709–714.

Levin, E. R., et al. The influence of pyridoxine in diabetic peripheral neuropathy. *Diabetes Care* (1981) 4:606–609.

Levy, G., and Leonards, J. Urine pH and salicylate therapy. *Journal of the American Medical Association* (1971) 217:81.

Lindenbaum, J. Drugs and vitamin B_{12} and folate metabolism. *Current Concepts in Nutrition* (1983) 12:73–87.

Livingstone, P. E., and Jones, C. Treatment of intermittent claudication with vitamin E. *Lancet* (1968) 2:602–603.

Livingstone, S., Berman, W., and Pauli, L. L. Anticonvulsant drugs and vitamin D metabolism. *Journal of the American Medical Association* (1973) 224:1634.

Lopez, R., Schwartz, J. V., and Cooperman, J. M. Riboflavin deficiency in an adolescent population in New York City. *American Journal of Clinical Nutrition* (1980) 33:1283–1286.

Luhby, A. L., et al. Vitamin B_6 metabolism in users of oral contraceptive agents. I: Abnormal urinary xanthurenic acid excretion and its correction by pyridoxine. *American Journal of Clinical Nutrition* (1971) 24:684–693.

MacDonald, H. N., Collins, Y. D. and Tobin, M.J.W. Failure of pyridoxine in suppression of puerteral lactation. *British Journal of Obstetric and Gynaecology* (1976) 83:54–55.

Mangini, R. J., ed. *Drug Interaction Facts.* St. Louis: Facts & Comparisons Division of J. B. Lippincott, 1984.

Manolagas, S. C., and Deftos, L. J. The vitamin D endocrine system and the hematolymphpoietic tissue. *Annals of Internal Medicine* (1984) 100:144–146.

Marks, J. *A Guide to the Vitamins.* Lancaster, England: Medical and Technical, 1976.

Marshall, J., et al. Diet in the epidemiology of oral cancer. *Nutrition and Cancer* (1982) 3:145–149.

Mason, R. S., et al. Vitamin D conversion by sarcoid lymph node homogenate. *Annals of Internal Medicine* (1974) 100:59–61.

Mattingly, P. C., et al. Zinc sulphate in rheumatoid arthritis. *Annals of Rheumatic Diseases* (1982) 41:456–457.

Matts, S.G.F. Riboflavin. In: *Vitamins in Medicine, Vol. 1,* ed.

B. M. Barker and D. A. Bender. London: Heinemann Medical Books, 1980.

Mayer, H., et al. Retinoids, a new class of compounds with prophylactic and therapeutic effects in oncology and dermatology. *Experientia* (1978) 340:1105–1246.

Meadows, G. G., et al. Amitriptyline related peripheral neuropathy relieved during pyridoxine hydrochloride administration. *Drug Intelligence and Clinical Pharmacy* (1982) 16:876–877.

McCarron, D. A. Calcium and magnesium nutrition in human hypertension. *Annals of Internal Medicine* (1983) 98:800–805.

McCarty, M. F., and Rubin, E. J. Rationales for micronutrient supplementation in diabetes. *Medical Hypotheses* (1984) 13:139–151.

McEvoy, A. W., et al. Vitamin B_{12} absorption does not decline with age in normal elderly humans. *Age and Aging* (1982) 11:180–183.

McMahon, F. G., et al. Upper gastrointestinal lesions after potassium chloride supplements: A controlled clinical trial. *Lancet* (1982) 2:1059–1061.

Mejia, L. A. Determination of vitamin A in blood. Some practical considerations in the time of collection of the specimens and stability of the vitamin. *American Journal of Clinical Nutrition* (1983) 37:147–151.

Mettlin, C., Graham, S. and Swanson, M. Vitamin A and lung cancer. *Journal of the National Cancer Institute* (1979) 62:1435–1438.

Mihaly, G. W., et al. High dose of antacid (Mylanta II) reduces bioavailability of ranitidine. *British Medical Journal* (1982) 285:998–999.

Miles, D. A. Functions of zinc: A literature resume. *Journal of Oral Medicine* (1982) 37:95–97.

Miller, J. C., et al. Therapeutic effect of vitamin C: A co-twin study. *Journal of the American Medical Association* (1977) 241:908.

Mimnaugh, E. G., et al. The effects of alpha-tocopherol on the toxicity, disposition and metabolism of adriamycin in mice. *Toxicology and Applied Pharmacology* (1979) 49:119–126.

Mitchel, H. S., et al. *Nutrition in Health and Disease*. 16th ed. New York: Lippincott, 1976.

Bibliography

Mock, D. M., et al. Biotin deficiency: An unusual complication of parenteral alimentation. *New England Journal of Medicine* (1981) 304:820–823.

Monsen, E. R., and Balintfy, J. L. The bioavailability of iron. *Journal of the American Dietetic Association* (1982) 80:307–311.

Moran, D. M., et al. Zinc deficiency dermatitis accompanying parenteral nutrition supplemented with trace elements. *Clinical Pharmacy* (1982) 1:169–176.

Moran, J. R., and Greene, H. L. The B vitamins and vitamin C in human nutrition. *American Journal of Disabled Children* (1979) 133:192–199.

Mudd, H. S. Pyridoxine responsive genetic disease. *Federation Proceedings* (1971) 30:970–976.

Neuman, J. L., et al. Riboflavin deficiency in women taking oral contraceptive agents. *American Journal of Clinical Nutrition* (1978) 31:247–249.

Newberne, P. M., and Suphakarn, V. Preventive role of vitamin A in colon carcinogenesis in rats. *Cancer* (1977) 40:2553–2556.

Nichols, B. L., and Nichols, V. N. Nutritional physiology in pregnancy and lactation. *Advances in Pediatrics* (1983) 30:473–515.

O'Connor, M. E., et al. Vitamin K deficiency and breast feeding. *American Journal of Disabled Children* (1983) 37:601–602.

Oderda, G. M. Iron and vitamin toxicities. *Ear Nose Throat Journal* (1983) 62:84–87.

Olson, J. A. Adverse effects of large doses of vitamin A and retinoids. *Seminars in Oncology* (1983) 10:290–293.

Olson, J. A., et al. The function of vitamin A. *Federation Proceedings* (1983) 42:2740–2746.

Omdahl, J. L. Nutritional status in a healthy elderly population: Vitamin D. *American Journal of Clinical Nutrition* (1982) 36:1225–1233.

Ophir, O., et al. Low blood pressure in vegetarians: The possible role of potassium. *American Journal of Clinical Nutrition* (1983) 37:755–762.

Oveson, L. Vitamin therapy in the absence of obvious deficiency. What is the evidence? *Drugs* (1984) 27:148–170.

Pal, B., and Mukherjie, S. Chromium in nutrition. *Journal of Applied Nutrition* (1978) 30:14–18.

Parfitt, A. M., et al. Vitamin D and bone health in the elderly. *American Journal of Clinical Nutrition* (1982) 36 (supp. 5):1014–1031.

Pauling, L. *Vitamin C and the Common Cold*. San Francisco: W. H. Freeman, 1970.

Pauling, L. *Vitamin C, the Common Cold and the Flu*. San Francisco: W. H. Freeman, 1976.

Peck, G. L. Retinoids: Therapeutic use in dermatology. *Drugs* (1982) 24:341–351.

Peck, G. L., et al. Prolonged remission of cystic and conglobate acne with 13-cis retinoic acid. *New England Journal of Medicine* (1979) 300:329–333.

Pennington, J. A. *Dietary Nutrient Guide*. Westport, Conn.: AUI, 1976.

Pennington, J. A. Total diet study results and plans for selected minerals in foods. *FDA By-lines* (1980) 4:179–188.

Perlman, I., et al. Night vision in a case of vitamin A deficiency due to malabsorption. *British Journal of Ophthalmology* (1983) 67:37–42.

Phelps, D. L. Vitamin E and retrolental fibroplastic in 1982. *Pediatrics* (1982) 70:420–425.

Pitt, H. A., and Costrini, A. M. Vitamin C prophylaxis in marine recruits. *Journal of the American Medical Association* (1979) 241:908.

Prasad, A. S. Zinc deficiency in human subjects. *Progress in Clinical Biology Research* (1983) 129:1–33.

Prasad, A. S. *Zinc in Human Nutrition*. Boca Raton, Fla.: CRC Press, 1979.

Prasad, A. S., and Oberleas, D., eds. *Trace Elements in Human Health and Disease*. New York: Academic Press, 1976.

Puklin, J. E., Simon, R. M., and Ehrenkrantz, R. A. Influence on retrolental fibroplasia of intramuscular vitamin E during respiratory distress syndrome. *Ophthalmology* (1982) 89:96.

Rasmussen, H. Cellular calcium metabolism. *Annals of Internal Medicine* (1983) 98:809–816.

Read, A. P., et al. Spina bifida and vitamins (letter). *British Medical Journal* (1983) 286:560–561.

Resnick, L. M., et al. Divalent cations in essential hypertension. Relations between serum ionized calcium, magnesium and plasma renin activity. *New England Journal of Medicine* (1983) 309:888–891.

Ritchie, J. H., et al. Edema and hemolytic anemia in premature infants. *New England Journal of Medicine* (1968) 279:1185–1190.

Rivlin, R. S. Misuse of hair analysis for nutritional assessment. *American Journal of Medicine* (1983) 75:489–493.

Roberts, H. J. Potential toxicity due to dolomite and bonemeal. *Southern Medical Journal* (1983) 76:556–559.

Robertson, L., Flinders, C., and Godfrey, B. *Laurel's Kitchen*. New York: Bantam Books, 1976.

Roe, D. A. Nutrient toxicity with excessive intake. *New York State Journal of Medicine* (1966) 66:869.

Rosenberg, L. E. Vitamin dependent genetic disease. *Hospital Practice* (1970) 5:59–66.

Rosenthal, G. Interaction of ascorbic acid and warfarin. *Journal of the American Medical Association* (1971) 215:1671.

Rowland, M. Amphetamine blood and urine levels in man. *Journal of Pharmaceutical Sciences* (1969) 58:508–509.

Rudman, D., and Williams, P. J. Megadose vitamins—use and misuse. *New England Journal of Medicine* (1983) 309:488–489.

Russell, R. M., et al. Zinc and the special senses. *Annals of Internal Medicine* (1983) 99:227–239.

Russell, R. M., and Naccarto, D. V. Current perspectives on trace elements. *Drug Therapy* (1982) 10:115–125.

Sandtead, H. H., et al. Zinc nutrition in the elderly in relation to taste acuity, immune response, and wound healing. *American Journal of Clinical Nutrition* (1982) 36:1046–1059.

Savage, D., et al. Relapses after interruption of cyanocobalamine therapy in patients with pernicious anemia. *American Journal of Medicine* (1983) 74:765–772.

Schaumberg, H., et al. Sensory neuropathy from pyridoxine abuse: A new megavitamin syndrome. *New England Journal of Medicine* (1983) 309:445–448.

Schnoes, H. K., and DeLuca, H. F. Recent progress in vitamin D metabolism and the chemistry of vitamin D metabolites. *Federation Proceedings* (1980) 39:2723–2724.

Schrasch, C. J., et al. Clinical effects of vitamin C in elderly inpatients with low blood vitamin C levels. *Lancet* (1979) 1:403–405.

Schrauzer, G. N., and White, D. A. Selenium in human nutrition: Dietary intakes and effects of supplementation. *Biological-Inorganic Chemistry* (1978) 8:303–318.

Schrauzer, G. N., White, D. A., and Schneider, C. J. Cancer mortality correlation studies. III: Statistical associations with dietary selenium. *Biological-Inorganic Chemistry* (1977) 7:23–24.

Schrauzer, G. N., White, D. A., and Schneider, C. J. Selenium and cancer: Effects of selenium and of the diet on the genesis of spontaneous mammary tumors in virgin inbred female C_3H/St mice. *Biological-Inorganic Chemistry* (1978) 8:387–396.

Scott, M. L. Advances in our misunderstanding of vitamin E. *Federation Proceedings* (1980) 39:2736–2739.

Scriver, C. R. Vitamin responsive errors of metabolism. *Metabolism* (1973) 22:1319–1344.

Sebrel, W. H., and Harris, W. H. *The Vitamins*. Vol. 5. New York: Academic Press, 1972.

Seelig, M. S. Vitamin D and cardiovascular, renal and brain damage in infancy and childhood. *Annals of the New York Academy of Science* (1969) 147:537–582.

Sestili, M. A. Possible adverse effects of vitamin C and ascorbic acid. *Seminar in Oncology* (1983) 10:299–304.

Shamoo, A. E., and Ambudkar, I. S. Regulation of calcium transport in cardiac cells. *Canadian Journal of Physiology and Pharmacology* (1984) 46:485–495.

Sharman, I. M., Down, M. G., and Norgan, N. G. The effects of vitamin E on physiological function and athletic performance of trained swimmers. *Sports Medicine* (1976) 16:215–223.

Shoden, R. J., and Griffith, W. S. *Fundamentals of Clinical Nutrition*. New York: McGraw-Hill, 1980.

Shohet, S. B., et al. Vitamin E and blood cell function. *Annals of the New York Academy of Science* (1983) 3:59–62.

Shute, W. E. *Vitamin E for Ailing and Healthy Hearts*. New York: Pyramid Press, 1972.

Silverman, J. E., et al. Zinc supplementation and taste in head and neck cancer patients undergoing radiation therapy. *Journal of Oral Medicine* (1983) 38:14–16.

Bibliography

Sjoquist, F., et al. The pH dependent excretion of monomethylates tricyclic antidepressants. *Clinical Pharmacology and Therapeutics* (1969) 10:826–833.

Slovik, D. M. The vitamin D endocrine system, calcium metabolism and osteoporosis. *Special Topics in Endocrinology and Metabolism* (1983) 5:83–148.

Smit, A. J., et al. Zinc deficiency during captopril treatment. *Nephron* (1983) 34:196–197.

Smith, A. H. Relationship between vitamin A and lung cancer. *National Cancer Institute Monograph* (1982) 62:165–166.

Smith, C. N. Repellants for anopheles mosquitos. *Miscellaneous Publications of the Entomology Society of America* (1970) 7:99–117.

Smith, G. F., et al. Failure of vitamin mineral supplementation in Down's syndrome (letter). *Lancet* (1983) 2:41.

Smith, I. J., et al. Vitamin E in retrolental fibroplasia (letter). *New England Journal of Medicine* (1983) 309:669.

Sokol, R. J. Vitamin E deficiency in adults (letter). *Annals of Internal Medicine* (1984) 100:769.

Sokol, R. J., et al. Vitamin E deficiency with normal serum vitamin E concentration in children with chronic cholestasis. *New England Journal of Medicine* (1984) 310:1209–1212.

Solomons, N. W., et al. Growth retardation and zinc nutrition. *Pediatric Research* (1976) 10:923–927.

Sommer, A. Increased mortality in children with mild vitamin A deficiency. *Lancet* (1983) 2:585–588.

Spencer, H., et al. Calcium requirements in humans: Report of original data and a review. *Clinical Orthopedics* (1984) 184:270–280.

Spencer, H., et al. Effect of small doses of aluminum containing antacids on calcium and phosphorous metabolism. *American Journal of Clinical Nutrition* (1982) 36:32–40.

Stadtman, T. C. Biological function of selenium. *Nutrition Review* (1977) 35:161–166.

Stamier, J., et al. Clofibrate and niacin in coronary heart disease. *Journal of the American Medical Association* (1975) 231:360–381.

Stern, H. J. Riboflavin treatment of spring catarrh. *American Journal of Ophthalmology* (1949) 32:1553–1555.

Strauss, W. G., et al. Drugs and disease as mosquito repellants in man. *American Journal of Tropical Medicine and Hygiene* (1968) 17:411–464.

Sugarman, A. A., and Clark, C. G. Jaundice following the administration of niacin. *Journal of the American Medical Association* (1979) 228:202.

Sugarman, B. Zinc and spinal cord injury: A review. *Journal of the American Paraplegia Society* (1984) 7:39–42.

Suttie, J. W. The metabolic role of vitamin K. *Federation Proceedings* (1980) 39:2730–2735.

Tang, R. C. The quandary of vitamin D in the newborn infant. *Lancet* (1983) 1:1370–1372.

Taylor, T. V., et al. Ascorbic acid supplementation in the treatment of pressure areas. *Lancet* (1974) 2:544–546.

Terezhalmy, G. T., et al. The use of water soluble bioflavinoid-ascorbic acid complex in the treatment of recurrent herpes labialis. *Oral Surgery, Oral Medicine, Oral Pathology* (1978) 45:56–62.

Ting, S., et al. Effects of ascorbic acid on pulmonary functions in mild asthma. *Journal of Asthma* (1983) 20:39–42.

Trader, J., Reibman, B., and Turkewitz, D. Vitamin B_{12} deficiency in strict vegetarians. *New England Journal of Medicine* (1978) 299:1319–1320.

Treasure, J., and Ploth, D. Role of dietary potassium in the treatment of hypertension. *Hypertension* (1983) 5:864–872.

Truesdell, D. D., Whitney, E. B., and Acosta, P. B. Nutrients in vegetarian foods. *Journal of the American Dietetic Association* (1984) 84:28–35.

Tuckerman, M. M., and Turco, S. J. *Human Nutrition.* Philadelphia: Lea and Febiger, 1983.

Underwood, E. J. *Trace Elements in Human and Animal Nutrition.* New York: Academic Press, 1977.

Vallely, J. F., Lovegrove, T. D., and Hobbs, G. E. Nicotinic acid and nicotinamide in the treatment of chronic schizophrenia. *Canadian Psychiatric Association Journal* (1971) 16:433–435.

Van Dam, B. Vitamins and sport. *British Journal of Sports Medicine* (1977) 12(2):74–79.

Vatassery, G. T., et al. Vitamin E concentrations in human

blood plasma and platelets. *American Journal of Clinical Nutrition* (1983) 37:1020–1024.

Victor, M. The Wernicke-Korsakoff syndrome: A clinical and pathological study of 245 patients, 82 with post-mortem examinations. *Contemporary Neurology* (1971) 7:1–206.

Vina, J., Hems, R., and Krebs, H. A. Reduction of formaminoglutamate with liver glutamate dehydrogenase. *Biochemistry Journal* (1978) 170:711–713.

Wade, A. E., et al. Effects of dietary thiamin intake on hepatic drug metabolism in the male rat. *Biochemical Pharmacology* (1969) 18:2288–2292.

Welsh, S. O., and Marston, R. M. Zinc in the U.S. food supply. *Food Technology* (January 1982): 70–76.

Whanger, A. Vitamins and vigor at 65 plus. *Postgraduate Medicine* (1973) 53:167–172.

Willett, W. C., and MacMahon, B. Diet and cancer—an overview. *New England Journal of Medicine* (1984) 310:633–638.

Willett, W. C., et al. Relation of vitamins A and E and carotenoids to the risk of cancer. *New England Journal of Medicine* (1984) 310:430–434.

Willett, W. C., et al. Selenium and cancer. *Lancet* (1983) 2:130–134.

Williams, H.T.G., Fenna, D., and Macbeth, R. A. Alpha tocopherol in the treatment of intermittent claudication. *Surgical Gynecology and Obstetrics* (1971) 132:662–666.

Wills, M. R., and Savory, J. Vitamin D metabolism and chronic liver disease. *Annals of Clinical Laboratory Science* (1984) 14:189–197.

Wilson, C.W.M., and Loh, H. S. Common cold and vitamin C. *Lancet* (1973) 1:638.

Winick, M. *Nutrition in Health and Disease*. New York: Wiley, 1980.

Winter, S. L., and Boyer, J. L. Hepatic toxicity from large doses of vitamin B_3 (nicotinamide). *New England Journal of Medicine* (1971) 20:1180–1182.

Yang, G., et al. Selenium toxicity in China. *American Journal of Clinical Nutrition* (1983) 37:872–881.

Zipursky, A., et al. Effect of vitamin E therapy on blood coagulation tests in newborn infants. *Pediatrics* (1980) 66:547–550.

Appendix:

VITAMIN AND MINERAL
CONTENT OF FOODS

How to Use These Tables

The following tables are meant to provide you with basic information on the amount of some important vitamins and minerals contained in the food we eat. Many foods are given more than one listing to represent amounts of vitamins and minerals contained in different forms of the same food. There are also listings for foods with different nutrient content before and after cooking. Be sure to select the listing that most closely approximates the type of food you are measuring and its form.

The information in the tables was gleaned from several sources, including U.S. Department of Agriculture publication no. 456, *Nutritive Value of American Foods*. This USDA publication does not contain data for all vitamins, minerals, and pseudovitamins. The job of analyzing and cataloguing that much information is too great even for the federal government! So we are left with a document that provides a massive amount of information on many of the vitamins as well as some minerals that have been recognized as being essential to human growth and function.

To use the charts and tables properly, you must keep an accurate record of the foods you eat every day. The food tables are divided into nine convenient categories: dairy products; fish and fowl (including eggs); fruits, grains, and grain products; meats; cold cuts, sausage, and luncheon meats; nuts; sugars, sweets, and desserts; vegetables; and miscellaneous foods. A special supplement to the tables lists the vitamin contents of various fast food products.

We have made a special effort to include, under other headings, a wide variety of food sources that also contain vitamins and minerals not listed in these tables. Most of these vitamins and minerals are available in a great variety of foods and are so widespread that most people do not have to think about obtaining sufficient quantities in their daily diet; others are controversial in terms of their basic application to human nutrition. However, food sources for vitamins and minerals not included here can be found in their individual profiles.

As you might expect, it is now possible to use your home computer to analyze the vitamin and mineral content of your diet. A number of programs that operate on standard personal computers such as Apple and IBM can be ordered from any computer store. Some are geared (and priced: $1000 and up!) for the professional who intends to use the program as part of a nutrition or diet counselling practice. Others are intended for home use and priced from $40 to $250. These programs ask you to tell them the kind and quantity of food eaten for a given period of time, usually a day or a week, and will give back an analysis of the nutrient content of those foods, telling you when nutrient supplements are needed. Several of the programs offer other, more sophisticated analyses, too.

Some of the more useful programs in this area are: *Dine* (about $75), *Health Aide* (about $80), *Nutrichec* (about $60), *Nutrient Trackor 15* (about $40) and *The Nutritionist* (about $150). Be sure to test any food analysis program before buying to be certain that it fills your needs.

DAIRY PRODUCTS

Item	Amount	Calories	Protein grams	Calcium mg.	Iron mg.	Sod mg.	Potass mg.	A mcg.	Thia mg.	Ribo mg.	Nia mg.	C mg.	B6 mg.	E mg.	Folic Acid mg.
Butter	1 tsp	36	0	1	0	49	1	165	0	0	0	0	0	0.1	0
Butter (whipped)	1.tsp	48	0	1	0	65	1	224	0	0	0	0	0	0.1	0
Butter Milk	1 cup	88	8.8	296	0.1	319	343	10	0.1	0.44	0.25	2.5	0.09	0.25	27
Natural Cheeses:															
Blue (Roquefort)	1 oz	103	6	88	0.14	186	22	347	0.01	0.17	0.3	0	0.05	0.2	3
Brick	1 oz	103	6	198	0.4	0	0	346	0.01	0.13	0.03	0	0.02	0	0
Camembert	1 oz	81	4.8	28	0.14	0	31	277	0.01	0.21	0.22	0	0.06	0	2
Cheddar	1 oz	111	7	210	0.3	196	23	367	0.01	0.13	0.1	0	0.02	0.4	31
Cottage Cheese	½ cup	121	15.5	107	0.3	261	24	194	0.03	0.29		0	0.05	0.1	4
Cream Cheese	1 oz	105	2.2	17	0.1	70	21	431	0.01	0.07	0	0	0.02	0.3	4
Cream Cheese (Whipped)	1 oz	104	2.2	17	0.1	70	21	214	0.01	0.07	0	0	0.02	0.3	4
Limburger	1 oz	96	5.9	165	0.17	0	0	318	0.02	0.14	0.06	0	0.02	0	0
Parmesan	1 oz	118	11	340	0.11	219	45	318	0.01	0.22	0.06	0	0.03	0	0
Swiss	1 oz	103	7.7	258	0.25	198	29	0	0	0.11	0.03	0	0.02	0	0
Cheese—Pasteurized Process:															
American	1 slice	70	4.4	132	0.2	216	15	342	0.01	0.08	0	0	0.02	0.3	3
American	1 oz	104	6.5	195	0.3	318	22	340	0.01	0.11	0	0	0.02	0.3	3
Swiss	1 slice	75	5.5	186	0.2	245	21	230	T	0.08	T	0	0.01	0.17	0
Swiss	1 oz	101	70	251	0.25	331	28	312	T	0.11	0.03	0	0.01	0.25	0

Item	Amount	Calories	Protein grams	Calcium mg.	Iron mg.	Sod mg.	Potass mg.	A mcg.	Thia mg.	Ribo mg.	Nia mg.	C mg.	B₆ mg.	E mg.	Folic Acid mg.
Cream:															
Half & Half	1 oz	41	0.96	33	0.01	14	39	145	0.01	0.05	0.01	0.3	0	0	0
Light Cream	1 oz	63	0.9	31	0.01	13	37	259	0.01	0.05	0.01	0.3	0.01	0	0
Heavy Cream	1 oz	105	0.65	22	0.01	10	27	459	T	0.03	0.01	0.3	0.01	0	0
Ice Cream	½ cup	186	3.6	111	0	36	101	468	0.04	0.17	0.1	1	0.03	0.1	1
Ice Milk	½ cup	144	3.5	116	0	35	107	220	0.05	0.18	0.1	1	0.03	0.1	1
Milk, Whole	1 cup	159	8.5	288	0.1	122	351	350	0.07	0.41	0.2	2	0.1	0.24	1.5
Milk, Skim	1 cup	88	8.8	296	0.1	127	355	10	0.09	0.44	0.2	2	0.1	0.24	0.3
Milk, Low Fat	1 cup	145	10.3	352	0.1	150	431	200	0.1	0.52	0.2	2	0.1	0.24	0
Yogurt (made from whole milk)	1 cup	152	7.4	272	0.1	115	323	340	0.07	0.39	0.2	2	0.1	0	0
Yogurt (made from partially skimmed milk)	1 cup	123	8.3	294	0.1	125	350	170	0.1	0.44	0.02	2	0.11	0	0
EGGS, FISH AND FOWL															
Bass, Sea	3 oz	216	135		0	0	0	42							
Bass, Sea—ovenfried and breaded	3 oz	165	18		0	0	0								
Blue Fish baked or broiled	3 oz	132	22	24.3	0.6	87			0.09	0.09	1.5				
Blue Fish fried	3 oz	171	19	29.4	0.8	120			0.09	0.09	1.5				

311

Item	Amount	Calories	Protein grams	Cal-cium mg.	Iron mg.	Sod mg.	Potass mg.	A mcg.	Thia mg.	Ribo mg.	Nia mg.	C mg.	B₆ mg.	E mg.	Folic Acid mg.
Caviar	1 oz	74	7.6	78	3.3	624	51								
Chicken															
light meat	3 oz	138	26.4	9.3	1	53	345	51	0.03	0.09	9.6	0	21	0.21	2.5
dark meat	3 oz	147	23.4	11	1.4	72	270	126	0.06	1.18	4.8	0	0.3	0.2	2.5
canned	3 oz	168	18.4	18	1.3	340	210	195	0.03	0.1	3.7	3	2.5	0.1	6.2
Chicken a La King	3 oz	159	9	45	0.9	258	138	390	0.03	0.15	1.8	4			
Chicken Fricassee	3 oz	135	13	5.1	0.9	129	117	60	0.03	0.06	0.2				
Chicken Pot Pie	3 oz	195	8.4	25.2	1.2	213	123	1113	0.09	0.09	1.5	2			
Clams	5 small or ½ cup	98	15.8	55	4.1	1010	184	110	0.01	0.11	1.1	11	80	0.3	3
Cod (cooked)	3 oz	141	24	25.8	0.9	93	351	150	0.06	0.09	2.5				
Eggs:															
Fried	1	86	5.5	24	1	135	56	570	0.04	0.12	T				
Hard Boiled	1	72	5.7	24	1	54	57	520	0.04	0.12	T				
Poached	1	72	5.7	24	1	119	57	520	0.04	0.12	T				
Scrambled	1	97	6.3	45	1	144	82	600	0.04	0.12	T				
Fish Sticks	1	50	4.7	3	0.1				0.1	0.02	0.5				

Flounder	3 oz	172	25.5	29	1.2	202	500		0.06	0.07	2.1	2	0.14		
Halibut (broiled)	3 oz	145	21.4	14	0.7	114	211	578	0.04	0.06	7.1	3	289	0.5	14
Herring, smoked	1 fillet	84	8.9	26	0.6			10		0.11	1.3		0.06		36
Lobster meat	3 oz	78	15	54	0.6	177	150		0.09	0.06					
Lobster Newburgh	1 cup	485	26.5	218	2.3	573	428		0.18	0.28					
Mackerel (broiled)	3 oz	197	18	5	1	0	0	144	0.12	0.2	6.4	0	0.5	1.3	0
Perch (fried)	3 oz	189	16	28	1.1	129	237	0	0.09	0.09	1.5	0	0	0	0
Oysters	1 cup	158	20.2	226	13.2	175	290	740	0.34	0.43	6	0.1	0	0	.0
Rockfish (steamed)	3 oz	90	15	0	0	57	372	0	0.03	0.09	0	0.9	0	0	0
Roe (herring)	3 oz	99	18	12	1	0	0	0	0	0	0	1.8	0.12	0	0
Salmon (chinook)	3 oz	177	15	129	8	0	306	192	0.03	0.12	6	0	0.24	0	5.7
Salmon (cohoe)	3 oz	129	17	207	0.75	294	285	66	0.03	0.15	6	0	0	0	0
Salmon Fillet (broiled or baked)	3 oz	155	23	68	1	99	377	136	0.14	0.05	8.3	4	255	1.2	6
Salmon (baked)	3 oz	150	18.4	12	1.2	114	435	161	0.18	0.07	10.8	4	1.2	595	6
Sardines (canned)	2 med size (1 oz)	57	6.7	122	0.8	230	165	62	0.01	0.06	1.5	0	50	0.2	9

Item	Amount	Calories	Protein grams	Calcium mg.	Iron mg.	Sod mg.	Potass mg.	A mcg.	Thia mg.	Ribo mg.	Nia mg.	C mg.	B₆ mg.	E mg.	Folic Acid mg.
Scallops (cooked)	3 oz	93	19.5	96	2.5	222	399	0	0	0	0	0	0	0	0
Shad (baked)	3 oz	173	20	20.7	0.5	68	325	27	0.11	0.22	7.4	0	0	0	0
Shrimp	3 oz	80	17.8	66	1.4	107	173	34	0.02	0.03	2.8	9	42	0.4	2
Shrimp (fried)	3 oz	192	10.6	32.7	0.9	183	169	26	0.03	0.03	1.7	6	51.6	0.5	1.7
Sturgeon (steamed)	45	7.5	11	0.56	30	66	00	0	0	0	0	0	0	0	0
Sturgeon (smoked)	1 oz	42	8.7	0	0	0	0	0	0	0	0	0	0	0	0
Sword fish, broiled	3 oz	138	22	21	0.9	0	0	1614	0.03	0.03	8.7	0	0	0	0
Tile Fish	3 oz	114	20												
Tuna (in oil)	3 oz	165	24	66	1.6	0	0	96	0.03	0.09	10	0	0.3	0.51	0
Tuna (in water)	3 oz	109	24	14	1.4	35	241	0	0	0.09	11.5	0	0	0	
Tuna Salad	1 cup	349	30	41	2.7	0	0	590	0.08	0.23	10.3	2	0	0	0
Turkey	3 oz	224	23	9	1.8	79	377	144	0.09	0.17	9.7	2	340	0.3	9
Turkey Pot Pie	1 piece	550	24.1	63	3.2	633	459	3090	0.26	0.3	5.8	5			
Whitefish (cooked)	1 oz	61	4.3	0	0.1	55	82	570	0.03	0.03	0.7	T			
Whitefish (smoked)	3 oz	129	17	18											

314

FAST FOODS

Item	Amount	Calories	Protein grams	Calcium mg.	Iron mg.	Sod mg.	Potass mg.	A mcg.	B12 mg.	Thia mg.	Ribo mg.	Nia mg.	C mg.	B6 mg.	E mg.	Folic Acid mg.
ARBY'S																
Roast Beef	1	350	22	80	3.6	880	—	—	—	0.3	0.34	5	—	—	—	—
Beef and Cheese	1	450	27	200	4.5	1220	—	—	—	0.38	0.43	6	—	—	—	—
Super Roast Beef	1	620	30	100	5.4	1420	—	—	—	0.53	0.43	7	—	—	—	—
Junior Roast Beef	1	220	12	40	1.8	530	—	—	—	0.15	0.17	3	—	—	—	—
Ham and Cheese	1	380	23	200	2.7	1350	—	—	—	0.75	0.34	5	—	—	—	—
Turkey Deluxe	1	510	28	80	2.7	1220	—	—	—	0.45	0.34	8	—	—	—	—
Club Sandwich	1	560	30	200	3.6	1610	—	—	—	0.48	0.43	7	—	—	—	—
BURGER CHEF																
Hamburger	1	244	11	45	2	—	208	114	0.26	0.17	0.16	2.7	1	0.16	—	—
Big Shef Sandwich	1	569	23	152	3.6	—	382	279	0.63	0.26	0.31	4.7	1	0.31	—	—
Cheeseburger	1	290	14	132	2.2	—	218	267	0.36	0.18	0.21	2.8	1	0.17	—	—
Double Cheeseburger	1	420	24	223	3.2	—	360	431	0.73	0.2	0.32	4.4	1	0.31	—	—
Fish Filet	1	547	21	145	2.2	—	271	400	0.1	0.23	0.22	2.7	1	0.04	—	—
French Fries (small)	1	250	2	9	0.7	—	473	0	0	0.07	0.04	1.7	12	—	—	—
(large)	1	351	3	13	0.9	—	661	0	0	0.1	0.06	2.4	16	—	—	—
Funmeal Feast	1	545	15	61	2.8	—	688	123	0.26	0.25	0.21	4.6	13	0.16	—	—
Hot Chocolate	1	198	8	271	0.7	—	436	288	0.79	0.93	0.39	0.3	2	0.1	—	—
Mariner Platter	1	734	29	63	3.3	—	996	2069	0.56	0.34	0.23	5.2	24	0.09	—	—
Rancher Platter	1	640	32	66	5.3	—	1237	1750	1	0.29	0.38	8.6	24	0.61	—	—
Shake (vanilla)	12 oz	380	13	497	0.3	—	622	387	1.77	0.1	0.66	0.5	0	0.1	—	—
(chocolate)	12 oz	403	10	449	1.1	—	762	292	1.07	0.16	0.76	0.4	0	0.1	—	—
Super Shef Sandwich	1	563	29	205	4.5	—	578	754	0.87	0.31	0.4	6	9	0.45	—	—
Top Shef Sandwich	1	661	41	194	5.4	—	612	273	1.16	0.35	0.47	8.1	0	0.56	—	—

Item	Amount	Calories	Protein grams	Cal-cium mg.	Iron mg.	Sod mg.	Potass mg.	A mcg.	B$_{12}$ mg.	Thia mg.	Ribo mg.	Nia mg.	C mg.	B$_6$ mg.	E mg.	Folic Acid mg.
CHURCH'S FRIED CHICKEN																
White Chicken	1 portion	327	21	94	1	498	186	160	—	0.1	0.18	7.2	T	—	—	—
Dark Chicken	1 portion	305	22	14	1.3	475	206	140	—	0.1	0.27	5.3	1	—	—	—
DAIRY QUEEN																
Brazier Cheese Dog	1	330	15	168	1.6	—	—	—	1.22	—	0.18	3.3	—	0.7	—	—
Brazier Chili Dog	1	330	13	86	2	—	—	—	1.29	0.15	0.23	3.9	11	0.17	—	—
Brazier Dog	1	273	11	75	1.5	—	—	—	1.05	0.12	0.15	2.6	11	0.08	—	—
Brazier Fries Small	1	200	2	T	0.4	—	—	T	—	0.06	T	0.08	3.6	0.16	—	—
Large	1	320	3	T	0.4	—	—	T	—	0.09	T	1.2	4.8	0.3	—	—
Brazier Onion Rings	1	300	6	20	0.4	—	—	T	—	0.09	0.17	0.4	2.4	0.08	—	—
Dilly Bar	1	240	4	100	0.4	—	—	100	0.5	0.06	0.14	T	T	—	—	—
DQ Banana Split	1	540	10	350	1.8	—	—	750	0.9	0.6	0.6	T	18	—	—	—
DQ Cone Small	1	110	3	100	T	—	—	100	0.4	0.3	0.14	0.8	T	—	—	—
Regular	1	230	6	200	T	—	—	300	0.6	0.09	0.26	T	T	—	—	—
Large	1	340	10	300	T	—	—	400	1.2	0.15	0.43	T	T	—	—	—
DQ Dip Cone Small	1	150	3	100	0.4	—	—	100	0.4	0.03	0.17	T	T	—	—	—
Regular	1	300	7	200	T	—	—	300	0.6	0.09	0.34	T	T	—	—	—
Large	1	450	10	300	0.4	—	—	400	0.9	0.12	0.51	T	T	—	—	—
DQ Float	1	330	6	200	T	—	—	100	0.6	0.12	0.17	T	T	—	—	—
DQ Freeze	1	520	11	300	T	—	—	200	1.2	0.15	0.34	T	T	—	—	—
DQ Parfait	1	460	10	300	1.8	—	—	400	1.2	0.12	0.43	T	T	—	—	—
DQ Sandwich	1	140	3	60	0.4	—	—	100	0.2	0.03	0.14	0.4	T	—	—	—
DQ Sundae Small	1	170	4	100	0.7	—	—	100	0.5	0.03	0.17	0.4	T	—	—	—
Regular	1	290	6	200	1.1	—	—	300	0.6	0.06	0.26	T	T	—	—	—
Large	1	400	9	300	1.8	—	—	400	1.2	0.09	0.43	0.4	T	—	—	—

	Amount													
		—	—	—	—	—	—	—	—	—	—	—	—	—
		—	—	—	—	—	—	—	—	—	—	—	—	—
DQ Malt Small	1	340	10	300	1.8	—	—	400	1.2	0.06	0.34	0.4	2	—
Regular	1	600	15	500	3.6	—	—	750	1.8	0.12	0.6	0.8	4	—
Large	1	840	22	600	5.4	—	—	750	2.4	0.15	0.85	1.2	6	0.16
Fish Sandwich	1	400	20	60	1	—	—	T	1.2	0.15	0.26	3	T	0.16
Fish Sandwich with Cheese	1	440	24	150	0.4	—	—	100	1.5	0.15	0.26	3	T	—
Frozen Dessert	1	180	5	150	T	—	—	100	0.6	0.09	0.17	T	T	—
Mr. Misty Float	1	440	6	200	T	—	—	100	0.6	0.12	0.17	T	T	—
Mr. Misty Freeze	1	500	10	300	T	—	—	200	0.12	0.15	0.34	T	T	—
Mr. Misty Kiss	1	70	0	T	T	—	—	T	T	T	T	T	T	—
Super Brazier Chili Dog	1	555	23	158	4	—	—	—	2.67	0.42	0.48	8.8	2	0.27
Super Brazier Dog	1	518	20	158	4.3	—	—	T	2.09	0.42	0.44	7	14	0.17
Super Brazier Dog with Cheese	1	593	26	297	4.4	—	—	—	2.34	0.43	0.48	8.1	14	0.18
JACK IN THE BOX														
Apple Turnover	1	411	4	11	1.4	352	69	T	0.17	0.23	0.12	2.5	T	0.03
Breakfast Jack	1	301	18	177	2.5	1037	190	442	1.1	0.41	0.47	5.1	3	0.14
Cheeseburger	1	310	16	172	2.6	877	177	338	0.87	0.27	0.21	5.4	1	0.12
French Fries	1 order	270	3	19	0.7	128	423	T	0.17	0.12	0.02	1.9	4	0.22
French Toast	1 order	537	15	119	3	1130	194	522	1.62	0.56	0.3	4.4	9	0.47
Hamburger	1	263	13	82	2.3	566	165	49	0.73	0.27	0.18	5.6	1	0.11
Jumbo Jack Hamburger	1	551	28	134	4.5	1134	492	246	2.68	0.47	0.34	11.6	4	0.3
Jumbo Jack Hamburger with Cheese	1	628	32	273	4.6	1666	499	734	3.05	0.52	0.38	11.3	5	0.31
Moby Jack Sandwich	1	455	17	167	1.7	837	246	240	1.1	0.3	0.21	4.5	1	0.12
Omelettes:														
Double Cheese	1	423	19	276	3.6	899	208	797	1.33	0.33	0.68	2.5	2	0.14
Ham and Cheese	1	425	21	260	4	975	237	766	1.44	0.45	0.7	3	1	0.18
Ranchero Style	1	414	20	278	3.8	1098	260	853	1.5	0.33	0.74	2.6	1	0.18
Onion Rings	1 order	351	5	26	1.4	318	109	488	0.26	0.24	0.12	3.1	T	0.07
Pancakes	1 order	626	16	105	2.8	1670	237	488	0.56	0.63	0.44	4.6	26	0.19
Regular Taco	1	189	8	116	1.2	460	264	356	0.5	0.07	0.08	1.8	T	0.14

Item	Amount	Calories	Protein grams	Cal-cium mg.	Iron mg.	Sod mg.	Potass mg.	A mcg.	B_{12} mg.	Thia mg.	Ribo mg.	Nia mg.	C mg.	B_6 mg.	E mg.	Folic Acid mg.
Scrambled Eggs	1 order	719	26	257	5	1110	635	694	1.31	0.69	0.56	5.2	12	0.34	—	—
Shakes:																
Chocolate	1	365	11	350	1.2	294	633	380	0.98	0.16	0.6	0.6	3	0.18	—	—
Strawberry	1	380	11	351	0.3	268	556	426	0.92	0.16	0.62	0.5	3	0.18	—	—
Vanilla	1	342	10	349	0.4	263	536	440	1.1	0.16	0.47	0.5	4	0.18	—	—
Super Taco	1	285	12	196	1.9	968	415	599	0.77	0.1	0.12	2.8	2	0.22	—	—
KENTUCKY FRIED CHICKEN																
Original recipe:																
Drum and Thigh	1 order	643	35	—	—	—	—	26	—	0.25	0.32	8.5	37	—	—	—
Wing and Rib	1 order	603	30	—	—	—	—	26	—	0.22	0.19	10	37	—	—	—
Wing and Thigh	1 order	661	33	—	—	—	—	26	—	0.24	0.27	8.4	37	—	—	—
Extra Crispy:																
Drum and Thigh	1 order	765	38	—	—	—	—	26	—	0.32	0.38	10.4	37	—	—	—
Wing and Rib	1 order	755	33	—	—	—	—	26	—	0.31	0.29	10.4	37	—	—	—
Wing and Thigh	1 order	812	36	—	—	—	—	26	—	0.31	0.35	10.3	37	—	—	—
Coleslaw	3 ounces	122	1	—	—	—	—	T	T	T	T	T	T	—	—	—
Corn	1 ear	169	5	—	—	—	—	162	T	0.12	0.07	1.2	3	—	—	—
Gravy	1 Tbsp	23	0	—	—	—	—	2	T	0.01	0.01	0.1	T	—	—	—
Mashed Potatoes	1 order	64	2	—	—	—	—	15	T	0.02	0.02	0.8	5	—	—	—
Rolls	1	61	2	—	—	—	—	4	—	0.1	0.04	1	0.3	—	—	—
McDONALD's																
Apple Pie	1	253	2	14	0.6	398	39	33	0.03	0.02	0.02	0.2	T	0.02	—	—
Big Mac	1	563	26	157	4	1010	237	530	1.8	0.39	0.37	6.5	2	0.27	—	—
Cheeseburger	1	307	15	132	2.4	767	156	345	0.91	0.25	0.23	3.8	2	0.12	—	—

Food	Amount													
Cherry Pie	1	260	2	12	0.6	427	35	114	0.01	0.03	0.02	0.4	T	0.02
Egg McMuffin	1	327	19	226	2.9	885	168	97	0.75	0.47	0.44	3.8	1	0.21
English Muffin, Buttered	1	186	5	117	1.5	318	71	164	0.02	0.28	0.49	2.6	1	0.04
Filet-o-Fish	1	432	14	93	1.7	781	150	42	0.82	0.26	0.2	2.6	1	0.1
French Fries (Regular Size)	1 order	220	3	9	0.6	109	564	16	0.02	0.12	0.02	2.3	13	0.22
Hamburger	1	255	12	51	2.3	520	142	82	0.81	0.25	0.18	4	2	0.12
Hashbrowns	1 order	125	2	5	0.4	325	247	13	0.01	0.06	T	0.8	4	0.13
Hot Cakes with Butter and Syrup	1 order	500	8	103	2.2	1070	187	257	0.19	0.26	0.36	2.3	5	0.12
McDonald Land Cookies	1 box	308	4	12	1.5	358	52	26	0.03	0.23	0.23	2.9	1	0.03
Quarter Pounder	1	424	24	63	4.1	735	322	133	1.88	0.32	0.28	6.5	1	0.27
Quarter Pounder with Cheese	1	524	30	219	4.3	1236	341	660	2.15	0.31	0.37	7.4	3	0.23
Sausage Patty (Pork)	1	209	9	16	0.8	615	127	30	0.53	0.27	0.11	2.1	T	0.18
Scrambled Eggs	1 order	180	13	61	2.5	205	135	652	0.93	0.08	0.47	0.2	1	0.19
Shakes:														
Chocolate	1	383	10	320	0.8	300	580	349	1.16	0.12	0.44	0.5	2	0.13
Strawberry	1	362	9	322	0.2	207	423	377	1.16	0.12	0.44	0.4	4	0.14
Vanilla	1	352	9	329	0.2	201	422	349	1.19	0.12	0.7	0.3	3	0.12
Sundaes:														
Caramel	1	328	7	200	0.2	195	338	279	0.6	0.07	0.31	1	4	0.05
Hot Fudge	1	310	7	215	0.6	175	410	230	0.07	0.07	0.31	1.1	3	0.13
Strawberry	1	289	7	174	0.4	96	290	230	0.6	0.07	0.3	1	3	0.08
TACO BELL														
Bean Burrito	1	343	11	98	2.8	272	235	1657	—	0.37	0.22	2.2	15	—
Beef Burrito	1	466	30	83	4.6	327	320	1675	—	0.3	0.39	7	15	—
Beefy Tostada	1	291	19	208	3.4	138	277	3450	—	0.16	0.27	3.3	13	—
Bell Beefer	1	221	15	40	2.6	231	183	2961	—	0.15	0.2	3.7	10	—
Bell Beefer with Cheese	1	278	19	147	2.7	330	195	3146	—	0.16	0.27	3.7	10	—
Burrito Supreme	1	457	21	121	3.8	367	350	3462	—	0.33	0.35	4.7	16	—
Combination Burrito	1	404	21	91	3.7	300	278	1666	—	0.34	0.31	4.6	15	—
Enchirito	1	454	25	259	3.8	1175	491	1178	—	0.31	0.37	4.7	10	—

Item	Amount	Calories	Protein grams	Calcium mg.	Iron mg.	Sod mg.	Potass mg.	A mcg.	B₁₂ mg.	Thia mg.	Ribo mg.	Nia mg.	C mg.	B₆ mg.	E mg.	Folic Acid mg.
Pintos 'n Cheese	1	168	11	150	2.3	102	307	3123	—	0.26	0.16	0.9	9	—	—	—
Taco	1	186	15	120	2.5	79	143	120	—	0.09	0.16	2.9	T	—	—	—
Tostada	1	179	9	191	2.3	101	172	3152	—	0.18	0.15	0.8	10	—	—	—
WENDY'S																
Chili	1 order	230	19	83	4.4	1065	—	1188	—	0.22	0.25	3.4	3	—	—	—
French Fries	4 oz order	330	5	16	1.2	112	—	40	—	0.14	0.07	3	6	—	—	—
Frosty		390	9	270	0.9	247	—	355	—	0.2	0.6	T	0.7	—	0	—
Hamburger (single)		470	26	84	5.3	774	—	94	—	0.24	0.36	5.8	T	—	—	—
Hamburger (double)		670	44	138	8.2	980	—	128	—	0.43	0.54	10.6	2	—	—	—
Hamburger (triple)		850	65	104	10.7	1217	—	220	—	0.47	0.6	14.7	2	—	—	—
Single with Cheese		580	33	228	5.4	1085	—	221	—	0.38	0.43	6.3	T	—	—	—
Double with Cheese		800	50	177	10.2	1414	—	439	—	0.49	0.75	11.4	2	—	—	—
Triple with Cheese		1040	72	371	10.9	1848	—	472	—	0.8	0.84	15.1	3	—	—	—
PIZZA HUT																
Thin 'n Crispy—Medium Size Pizza:																
Cheese—Standard	2 slices	340	19	500	3.6	900	190	600	—	0.45	0.51	4	T	—	—	—
Cheese—Super Style	2 slices	410	26	800	3.6	1100	196	750	—	0.53	0.6	4	T	—	—	—
Pepperoni—Standard	2 slices	370	19	400	3.2	1000	225	700	—	0.45	0.43	4	T	—	—	—
Pepperoni—Super Style	2 slices	430	23	550	3.6	1200	270	800	—	0.6	0.43	5	T	—	—	—
Pork with Mushroom—Standard	2 slices	380	21	120	4.5	1200	340	750	—	0.53	0.51	6	T	—	—	—
Pork with Mushroom—Super Style	2 slices	450	26	150	6.3	1400	400	750	—	0.6	0.6	6	1	—	—	—
Supreme	2 slices	400	21	400	4.5	1200	335	750	—	0.68	0.51	6	2	—	—	—
Super Supreme	2 slices	520	30	550	5.4	1500	415	1100	—	1	0.68	8	4	—	—	—

Thick and Chewy—Medium Size Pizza:														
Cheese—Standard	2 slices	390	24	600	4.5	800	290	800	0.75	1.19	8	T	—	—
Cheese—Super Style	2 slices	450	31	950	4.5	1000	295	1000	0.83	0.68	8	T	—	—
Pepperoni—Standard	2 slices	450	25	500	4.5	900	300	1500	0.83	0.68	5	T	—	—
Pepperoni—Super Style	2 slices	490	27	500	3.6	1200	315	1000	0.83	0.68	6	1	—	—
Pork with Mushroom—Standard Style	2 slices	430	27	400	5.4	1000	420	1000	0.9	0.6	11	2	—	—
Pork with Mushroom—Super Style	2 slices	500	30	550	6.3	1200	495	1000	0.9	0.68	12	2	—	—
Supreme	2 slices	480	29	550	5.4	1000	405	1000	0.9	0.77	10	4	—	—
Super Supreme	2 slices	590	34	550	6.3	1400	465	1000	1.2	0.94	12	4	—	—
BURGER KING														
Apple Pie	1	240	2	T	0.28	335	50	T	T	0.03	T	T	—	—
Cheeseburger	1	350	18	32	2.1	730	230	T	0.12	0.17	2	T	—	—
Double Cheeseburger	1	530	30	64	2.1	990	360	T	0.15	0.25	3	T	—	—
Double Whopper	1	850	44	16	3.5	1080	760	T	0.09	0.43	8	T	—	—
Double Whopper with Cheese	1	950	50	120	2.8	1535	730	T	0.09	0.43	8	T	—	—
French Fries	1 reg. order	210	3	T	0.3	230	380	T	0.06	T	0.8	2	—	—
Hamburger	1	290	15	T	2.1	525	240	T	0.15	0.17	2	T	—	—
Onion Rings	1 regular order	270	3	64	0.28	450	140	T	0.06	T	T	T	—	—
Shakes:														
Chocolate	1	340	8	200	T	280	340	T	0.12	0.25	T	T	—	—
Vanilla	1	340	8	240	T	320	210	T	0.15	0.34	T	T	—	—
Whopper	1	630	26	32	2.1	990	520	T	0.06	0.25	4	T	—	—
Whopper with Cheese	1	740	32	120	2.1	1435	590	T	0.12	0.34	3	T	—	—
Whopper Junior	1	370	15	T	1.4	560	280	T	0.23	0.17	3	T	—	—
Whopper Junior with Cheese	1	420	18	64	1.4	785	270	T	0.23	0.17	3	T	—	—

FRUITS

Item	Amount	Calories	Protein grams	Calcium mg.	Iron mg.	Sod mg.	Potass mg.	A mcg.	Thia mg.	Ribo mg.	Nia mg.	C mg.	B₆ mg.	E mg.	Folic Acid mg.
Applesauce:															
sweetened	1 cup	232	0.5	10	1.3	5.	166	100	0.05	0.03	0.1	3	0.06	0	0
unsweetened	1 cup	100	0.5	10	1.2	5.	190	100	0.05	0.02	0.1	2	0.06	0	0
Apricots:															
raw	½ pound	109	2.2	36	1.1	2.5	599	5755	0.07	0.09	1.3	22	0.15	1	5
whole canned in syrup	3 medium halves	86	0.6	11	0.3	1	234	1740	0.02	0.02	0.4	4	0	0	0
whole canned in water	3 medium halves	38	0.7	12	0.3	1	246	1830	0.02	0.02	0.4	4	0	0	0
dehydrated, uncooked	17 large halves	260	5	67	5.5	26	979	10900	0.01	0.16	3.3	12	0	0	0
Apricot Nectar	1 cup	143	0.8	23	0.5	T	379	2380	0.03	0.03	0.5	8	0	0	0
Banana (raw)	1 medium	101	1.3	10	0.8	1	440	190	0.05	0.06	0.7	10	0.5	0.7	11
Blackberries															
raw	1 cup	84	1.7	46	1.3	1	245	200	0.03	0.03	0.4	21	0.1	4.5	37
canned	1 cup	135	2	63	2.3	2.5	425	350	0.05	0.05	0.5	2	0	0	0
Blueberries															
raw	1 cup	99	1.1	24	1.6	1.6	130	160	0.05	1	0.8	22	0.04	0	113
frozen	1 cup	88	1.1	16	1.3	1.6	130	112	0.05	1	0.8	11	0.09	0	0
Cantaloupe	¼ melon	30	0.7	14	0.4	12	251	3400	0.04	0.03	6	33	0.08	0.1	T

Casaba Melon	¼ melon	92	4.1	48	1.4	41	854	178	0.14	0.1	2	44	0	0	0
Cherries: sweet, raw	15 large or 25 small	70	1.3	22	0.4	2	191	110	0.05	0.06	0.4	10	0.04	0	0
raw	1 cup	116	2.4	44	0.8	4	382	220	0.1	0.12	0.8	21	0.14	0	0
Coconut meat	1 cup	780	8	30	3.8	52	581	0	0.12	0.04	1.2	7	0.1	2	62
Cranberries	1 cup	46	0.4	14	0.5	2	82	40	0.03	0.02	0.1	11	0.03	0	2
Cranberry Juice Cocktail	1 cup	165	0.25	13	0.75	2.5	25	T	0.03	0.03	T	41	0	0	0
Cranberry Sauce	5½ Tbsp.	146	0.1	6	0.2	1	30	4	T	T	T	2	0	0	0
Dates (whole without pits)	10 medium	274	2.2	59	0.3	1	648	50	0.09	1	2.2	0	0.17	0	28
Figs, whole	2 large/3 small	80	1.2	35	0.6	2	194	80	0.06	0.05	0.4	2	0.12	0	7
Fruit Cocktail	1 cup	91	1	22	1	12	412	150	0.02	0.01	0.5	2	0.08	0	0
Grapefruit: fresh	½ medium	41	0.5	16	0.4	1	135	10	0.04	0.02	0.2	38	0.06	0	4
sections	1 cup	87	1	61	0.8	2	257	20	0.08	0.04	0.4	76	0.06	0	0
juice	1 cup	96	1.2	22	0.5	2	399	200	0.1	0.05	0.5	93	0.27	0	0
Grapefruit/Orange Juice	1 cup	106	1.5	25	0.7	2	454	250	0.12	0.05	0.5	84	0.05	0	0
Grape: drink	1 cup	135	0.3	8	0.3	3	88	0	0.03	0.03	0.3	40	0	0	0
juice	1 cup	167	0.5	28	0.8	5	293	0	0.1	0.05	0.5	T	0	0	0
regular	10 grapes	45	0.4	8	0.3	2	115	70	0.03	0.02	0.2	3	0.06	0.5	4
seedless	10 grapes	34	0.3	6	0.2	2	87	50	0.03	0.02	0.2	2	0.06	0.5	4

Item	Amount	Calories	Protein grams	Calcium mg.	Iron mg.	Sod mg.	Potass mg.	A mcg.	Thia mg.	Ribo mg.	Nia mg.	C mg.	B₆ mg.	E mg.	Folic Acid mg.
Honeydew Melon	¼ melon	40	40	30	0.6	23	251	40	0.4	0.3	0.6	23	0.8	0.6	29
Lemon, raw	1 wedge	5	0.2	5	0.1	T	26	T	0.01	T	T	10	0.13	0	0
juice	1 cup	61	1.2	17	0.5	2	344	50	0.07	0.02	0.2	112	0.11	0	0
Lime, raw	1 wedge	19	0.5	5	0.4	1	69	10	0.02	0.01	0.1	25	0	0	0
juice	1 cup	64	0.7	22	0.5	2	256	20	0.05	0.02	0.2	79	0.1	0	0
Mango	1 fruit	152	1.6	23	0.9	16	437	11090	0.12	2.5	81		0	0	0
Orange:															
juice (canned)	1 cup	120	2	25	1	2	496	500	0.07	0.05	0.7	100	0.12	0	30
juice (fresh)	1 cup	112	1.7	27	0.5	2	496	500	0.22	0.07	1	124	0.08	0	10
juice (frozen)	1 cup	122	1.7	25	0.2	2	503	540	0.23	0.03	0.9	120	0.07	0	0
whole	1 fruit	71	1.8	56	0.6	1	271	280	0.14	0.06	0.6	85	0.12	0.4	10
Papaya	1 fruit	119	1.8	61	0.9	9	711	5320	0.12	0.12	0.9	170	0	0	0
Peaches:															
canned in syrup	1 cup	200	1	10	0.8	5	333	1100	0.03	0.05	1.5	8	0	0	0
canned in water	1 cup	76	1	10	0.7	5	334	1100	0.02	0.07	1.5	7	0.45	0	4
dried	1 cup	419	5	77	9.6	26	1520	6240	0.02	0.3	8.5	29	0	0	0
raw	1 fruit	51	0.8	12	0.7	1	269	1770	0.03	0.07	1.3	9	0.04	0	4
Peach Nectar	1 cup	120	0.5	10	0.5	2	194	1070	0.02	0.05	1	T	0	0	0

Food	Measure														
Pears:															
canned in syrup	1 cup	194	0.5	13	0.5	3	214	10	0.03	0.05	0.3	3	0	0	0
canned in water	1 cup	78	0.5	12	0.5	2	215	10	0.02	0.05	0.2	2	0	0	0
dried	1 cup	482	5.6	63	2.3	13	1031	130	0.02	0.32	1.1	13	0.34	0	0
raw	1 fruit	100	1.1	13	0.5	3	213	30	0.03	0.07	0.2	7	0.003	0.9	4
Pear Nectar	1 cup	130	0.8	8	0.3	3	98	T	T	0.05	T	T	0	0	0
Pineapple:															
canned in water	1 slice	78	0.3	12	0.3	0.1	101	50	0.08	0.02	2	1	0	0	0
juice, canned unsweetened	1 cup	138	1	4	0.1	T	373	130	0.13	0.05	0.5	23	0	0	0
juice, frozen	1 cup	130	1	28	0.8	3	340	30	0.13	0.05	0.5	30	0	0	0
raw	1 cup	206	0.6	28	0.8	2	234	112	0.14	0.04	0.4	28	0.15	1	2
Plums															
canned in syrup	1 cup	214	1	23	2.3	3	367	3130	0.05	0.05	1	5	0	0	0
canned in water	1 cup	114	1	22	2.5	5	368	3110	0.05	0.05	1	5	0	0	0
raw	1 fruit	32	0.3	8	0.3	1	112	160	0.02	0.02	0.3	4	0	0	0
Prunes, dried with pits	½ pound	579	4.8	116	8.5	18	1574	3630	0.2	0.39	3.7	7	0	0	11
Prune juice	1 cup	197	1	4	10.6	5	602	0	0.03	0.03	1	5	0	0	0
Pumpkin (canned)	1 cup	81	2.5	61	1	5	588	15680	0.07	0.12	1.5	12	0.25	0	0
Raisins:															
raw, whole	1 cup	419	3.6	90	5.1	39	1106	30	0.16	0.12	0.7	1	0.22	0	14
cooked with sugar	1 cup	628	3.5	86	4.7	38	1047	30	0.12	0.09	0.6	T	0	0	0
Raspberries:															
Black, raw	1 cup	98	2	40	1.2	1	267	T	0.04	0.12	1.2	24	0.27	0	0
Red, canned	1 cup	85	1.7	36	1.5	2	277	220	0.02	0.1	1.2	22	20	0	0

Item	Amount	Calories	Protein grams	Cal-cium mg.	Iron mg.	Sod mg.	Potass mg.	A mcg.	Thia mg.	Ribo mg.	Nia mg.	C mg.	B₆ mg.	E mg.	Folic Acid mg.
Red, frozen	1 cup	245	1.8	33	1.5	3	250	180	0.05	0.15	1.5	53	0	0	0
Red, raw	1 cup	70	1.5	27	1.1	1	207	160	0.04	0.11	1.1	31	0	20	23
Rhubarb, cooked with sugar added	1 cup	381	1.4	211	1.6	5	548	220	0.05	0.14	0.8	16	0	0	0
Strawberries:															
frozen	1 cup	278	1.3	36	1.8	3	286	80	0.05	0.15	1.3	135	0.1	0	0
raw	1 cup	56	1	32	1.5	2	246	90	0.04	0.1	0.9	88	0.08	0.3	7
Tangerine															
juice-unsweetened	1 cup	106	1.2	44	0.5	2	440	1040	0.15	0.05	0.2	54	0.007	0	0
juice-sweetened	1 cup	125	1.2	44	0.5	2	440	1040	0.15	0.05	0.2	54	0.007	0	0
juice-frozen	1 cup	114	1.2	45	0.5	2	432	1020	0.14	0.04	0.3	67	0	0	0
raw fruit	1 fruit	39	0.7	34	0.3	0.2	108	360	0.05	0.02	0.1	27	0	0	0
Watermelon	1 cup	41	0.8	11 16	0.8	0.8	2	158	0.05	0.05	0.3	11	0.11	0	30

GRAINS AND GRAIN PRODUCTS

Item	Amount	Calories	Protein grams	Calcium mg.	Iron mg.	Sod mg.	Potass mg.	A mcg.	Thia mg.	Ribo mg.	Nia mg.	C mg.	B₆ mg.	E mg.	Folic Acid mg.
Biscuit (homemade)	1	103	2.1	3.4	0.4	175	33	T	0.06	0.06	0.5	T			
Biscuit (from mix)	1	91	2.0	19	0.6	272	32	T	0.08	0.07	0.6	T			
Bran Flakes	1 cup	106	3.6	19	12.4	207	137	1650	0.41	0.49	0.41	12	0.39		
Breads:															
Cracked Wheat	1 slice	66	2.2	22	0.3	132	34	T	0.03	0.02	0.3	T	0.23		0.06
French Bread	1 slice	58	1.8	9	0.4	116	1	0	0.06	0.09	0.5	0	0.10	0	0.2
Italian	1 slice	54	1.8	16	0.4	117	15	0	0.06	0.04	0.05	0	0.09	0	0.2
Raisin Bread	1 slice	66	1.7	18	0.3	91	58	0	0.1	0.02	0.02	T			
Rye Bread	1 slice	61	2.3	19	0.4	139	36	0	0.05	0.02	0.4	0	0.25	0.73	4.0
Pumpernickel	1 slice	79	2.8	27	0.8	182	145	0	0.07	0.04	0.4	T	0.04	0.98	
White	1 slice	76	2.4	24	0.7	142	29	T	0.07	0.06	0.7	T			
Whole Wheat	1 slice	61	2.6	25	0.8	132	68	T	0.06	0.03	0.7	T	0.45		
Corn Bread	1 piece	161	5.8	94	0.9	490	122	120	0.1	0.15	0.5	1			
Crackers:															
Butter	10 crackers	151	2.3	49	0.2	360	37	70	T	0.01	0.3	0			
Cheese	10 crackers	44	1.0	3*	0.1	95	10	30	T	0.01	0.1	0			
Graham	1 large	55	1.1	6	0.2	95	55	0	0.01	0.03	0.2	0			
Saltines	10 crackers	123	2.6	6	0.3	312	34	0	T	0.01	0.3	0			
Soda	10 crackers	33	0.7	2	0.1	83	9	0	T	T	0.1	0			
Macaroni (enriched)	1 cup	192	6.5	14	1.4	1	103	0	0.23	0.13	0.18				

Item	Amount	Calories	Protein grams	Calcium mg.	Iron mg.	Sod mg.	Potass mg.	A mcg.	Thia mg.	Ribo mg.	Nia mg.	C mg.	B₆ mg.	E mg.	Folic Acid mg.
Macaroni & Cheese (cooked)	1 cup	430	16.8	362	1.8	1086	240	860	0.2	0.4	0.18				
Muffins from mix (homemade)	1	130	2.8	96	0.6	192	44	100	0.07	0.08	0.6	T			
Muffins (Blueberry)	1	112	2.9	34	0.6	253	46	90	0.06	0.08	0.5	T			
Muffins (Bran)	1	104	3.1	57	1.5	179	172	90	0.06	0.1	1.6	T			
Noodles (cooked)	1 cup	200	6.6	16	1.4	3	70	110	0.22	0.13	1.9	T			
Oatmeal, Instant (cooked)	1 cup	166	6.2	24	1.4	257	0	0	0.14	0	0	T	11.5		
Oatmeal, Regular (cooked)	1 cup	132	4.8	22	1.4	523	146	0	0.19	0.5	0.2	T			
Pancakes (from mix)	1	61	1.9	58	0.3	152	42	70	0.04	0.06	0.2	T			
Pastina (egg)	1 cup	651	21.9	60	4.9	9	9	370	1.5	0.65	10.2	T			
Popovers (homemade)	1	90	3.5	38	0.6	88	60	130	0.06	0.1	0.4	T			
Rice, long-grained brown (cooked)	1 cup	232	4.9	23	1	550	137	0	0.18	0.04	2.7	T	1.1	4.8	41.8
Rice, instant white (cooked)	1 cup	180	3.6	21	1.8	767	57	0	0.23	0.02	2.1	T	0.34	1.2	
Rice Pudding with Raisins	1 cup	387	9.5	260	1.1	188	469	290	0.08	0.37	0.5	T			

Item	Amount	Calories	Protein grams	Cal-cium mg.	Iron mg.	Sod mg.	Potass mg.	A mcg.	Thia mg.	Ribo mg.	Nia mg.	C mg.	B₆ mg.	E mg.	Folic Acid mg.
Rolls (home baked)	1	119	2.9	16	0.7	98	41	30	0.09	0.09	0.8	T	0.12		
Rolls (hard)	1	156	4.9	24	0.4	313	49	T	0.03	0.05	0.4	T			
Roll or Bun for frankfurter or hamburger	1	119	3.3	30	0.8	202	38	T	0.11	0.07	0.9	T			
Rye Wafers	10	224	8.5	34	2.5	573	390	T	0.21	0.16	0.8	T			
Salt Sticks	1	106	3.3	16	0.3	548	33	T	0.02	0.03	0.3	T			
Spaghetti (cooked)	1 cup	166	5	12	1	2	92	0	0.2	1.2	1.6	0	30	0	4
Waffle (homemade)	1	209	7	85	1.3	356	109	250	0.13	0.19	1.0	T			
Waffle (frozen)	1	86	2.4	41	0.6	219	54	40	0.06	0.05	0.4	T			
Waffle (from mix)	1	206	6.6	179	1	515	146	170	0.11	0.17	0.7	T			
Zwieback	1 piece	30	0.7	1	T	18	11	T	T	T	0.1				

MEATS

Item	Amount	Calories	Protein grams	Cal-cium mg.	Iron mg.	Sod mg.	Potass mg.	A mcg.	Thia mg.	Ribo mg.	Nia mg.	C mg.	B₆ mg.	E mg.	Folic Acid mg.
Bacon, Cooked	2 slices	86	3.8	2	0.5	155	35	0	0.08	0.05	0.8	0			
Bacon, Canadian	1 slice	58	5.7	3	0.9	537	91	0	0.19	0.04	1.1	0			

Item	Amount	Calories	Protein grams	Calcium mg.	Iron mg.	Sod mg.	Potass mg.	A mcg.	Thia mg.	Ribo mg.	Nia mg.	C mg.	B₆ mg.	E mg.	Folic Acid mg.
Beef:															
Boneless for Stew	¼ lb	371	29.5	13	3.8	52	236	50	0.06	0.22	4.5	0			
Chuck Roast or Steak	¼ lb	400	18.4	10	2.7	64	294	70	0.08	0.17	4.4	0			
Flank Steak	¼ lb	222	34.6	16	4.3	61	277	13	0.06	0.26	5.2	0			
Loin or Short Loin:															
Porterhouse	¼ lb	527	22.4	10	2.9	55	250	85	0.07	0.18	4.8	0			
T-Bone Steak	¼ lb	537	22.1	9	3	54	248	85	0.06	0.18	4.7	0			
Rib Roast	¼ lb	499	22.7	10	3	55	253	88	0.06	0.17	4.1	0			
Round Steak	¼ lb	296	32.2	14	4	90	363	30	0.09	0.25	6.3	0	0.4	0.3	4
Hamburger	¼ lb	248	31.1	14	4	76	348	23	0.1	0.26	6.8	0	0.5	0.4	5
Hamburger-Lean	¼ lb	324	27.5	14	3.6	67	308	43	0.1	0.24	6.1	0	0.5	0.4	5
Corned Beef (cooked)	¼ lb	422	26	10	3.3	1069	68	T	0.02	0.21	1.7	0	0.1	0.1	4
Chile Con Carne with Beans-Canned	1 cup	298	16.8	72	3.8	1189	522	134	0.07	0.16	2.9	4	0.2	0.4	20
Lamb:															
Leg of Lamb	¼ lb	317	29	13	1.9	70	322	T	0.17	0.31	6.23	0	0.31		4
Lamb Chops-Loin	1 chop	18	2.6	1	0.2	6	30	T	0.01	0.03	0.6	0			
Lamb Chops-Rib	1 chop	17	2.2	1	0.2	6	25	T	0.01	0.02	0.5	0			
Liver:															
Beef	¼ lb	260	30.0	12.5	10.0	209	431	60555	0.30	4.75	18.7	31	0.95	2.0	326
Calf	¼ lb	296	33.5	14.8	16.1	134	14	37083	0.27	4.73	18.7	42	0.75	1.5	329
Chicken	¼ lb	187	30.0	12.5	9.7	69	171	14198	0.19	3.05	13.3	18	0.85	1.8	427

Pork:	Amount	Calories	Protein grams	Calcium mg.	Iron mg.	Sod mg.	Potass mg.	A mcg.	Thia mg.	Ribo mg.	Nia mg.	C mg.	B6 mg.	E mg.	Folic Acid mg.
Ham-Cooked	¼ lb	424	26.0	11.3	3.4	64	292		T	0.58	0.26	5.2	0	0.36		8.8
Ham-Cooked Lean	¼ lb	246	33.7	15	4.3	83	377		T	0.73	0.33	6.5	0	0.45		11
Loin and Loin Chops (lean) baked or roasted	¼ lb	288	33.4	15	4.3	82	374		T	1.23	0.35	7.4	0	0.45		11
Spareribs Cooked	¼ lb	499	23.6	10	3.0	42	189		T	0.49	0.24	3.9				

SAUSAGE, COLD CUTS AND LUNCH MEATS

Item	Amount	Calories	Protein grams	Calcium mg.	Iron mg.	Sod mg.	Potass mg.	A mcg.	Thia mg.	Ribo mg.	Nia mg.	C mg.	B6 mg.	E mg.	Folic Acid mg.
Bockwurst	3 oz	228	9.7												
Boiled Ham	3 oz	202	16	9.5	2.4				0.12	0.04	0.71				
Bologna	3 oz	262	10.4	6	1.5	1120	198		0.04	0.06	0.71				
Braunschleiger (smoked liverwurst)	3 oz	275	12.7	8.5	5			1777	0.05	0.4	2.2				
Brown 'n Serve Sausage	3 oz	364	14.2												
Capicola	3 oz	430	17.4												
Country Style Sausage	3 oz	297	13	7.8	2				0.06	0.05	0.85				

Item	Amount	Calories	Protein grams	Calcium mg.	Iron mg.	Sod mg.	Potass mg.	A mcg.	Thia mg.	Ribo mg.	Nia mg.	C mg.	B₆ mg.	E mg.	Folic Acid mg.
Deviled Ham	3 oz	302	12	6.8	1.8				0.04	0.03	0.44				
Frankfurter:															
raw 5" long	1	176	7.1	4	1.1	627	125		0.09	0.11	1.5		B_6 0.14		
cooked 5" long	1	170	6.9	3	0.8				0.08	0.11	0.08				
Knockwurst	1 link	189	9.6	1.4	0.37				0.12	0.01	0.11				
	3 oz	340	12.2	6.8	1.8				0.05	0.06	0.71				
Liverwurst (fresh)	3 oz	265	14	7.8	4.6			1728	0.05	0.35	1.55		0.05	0.08	
Meat Loaf	3 oz	172	13.7	7.8	1.6				0.04	0.09	0.68				
Mortadella	1 slice	79	5.1	3	0.8										
	3 oz	272	17.6	10.3	2.7										
Polish Sausage	3 oz	262	13.5	7.8	2				0.09	0.05	0.85				
Pork Sausage (cooked)	1 link	62	2.4	1	0.3	125	35		0.01	0	0.5		0.01		
Salami	3 oz	388	20.5	12.2	3.1				0.1	0.07	1.44		0.03		0.72
Scrapple	3 oz	185	7.6	4.4	1				0.24	0.1	2.3				
Summer Sausage	3 oz	265	16	9.5	2.4				0.03	0.07	1.15		0.05		
Vienna Sausage (canned)	1 link	38	2.2	1	0.3				0	0	0.02		0		

MISCELLANEOUS FOODS

Item	Amount	Calories	Protein grams	Calcium mg.	Iron mg.	Sod mg.	Potass mg.	A mcg.	Thia mg.	Ribo mg.	Nia mg.	C mg.	B6 mg.	E mg.	Folic Acid mg.
Coffee (beverage)	1 cup	2	T	4	0.2	2	65	0	0	T	0.5	0	T	0	0
Hot Chocolate	1 cup	288	8.3	260	0.5	120	370	360	0.08	0.4	0.3	3	0	0	0
Jam and Preserves	1 Tbsp.	54	0.1	4	0.2	2	18	T	T	T	T	T	0	0	0
Maple Syrup	1 cup	794	0	328	3.8	32	554	0	0	0.1	0	0	0	0	0
Margarine:															
regular	1 Tbsp.	102	0.1	3	0	140	3	469	0	0	0	0	0	8	0
whipped	1 Tbsp.	68	0.06	0.9	0	93	2	313	0	0	0	0	0	5	0
Marmalade	1 Tbsp	51	0.1	7	0.1	3	7	0	T	T	T	1	0	0	0
Mustard:															
brown	1 Tbsp	14	0.9	19	0.3	196	20	0	0	0	0	0	0	0	0
yellow	1 Tbsp	11	0.7	13	0.3	188	20	0	0	0	0	0	0	0	0
Nuts:															
Almonds	2 Tbsp	195	6	76	1.5	1	—	0	0.08	0.3	1.2	T	0.06	0	288
Brazil Nuts (shelled)	2 Tbsp	239	3.9	50.6	0.9	30	195	0	0.3	0.03	0.44	0	0.04	4.7	T
Cashews	2 Tbsp	152	4.7	10.3	1	4	126	27	0.12	0.07	0.5	0	0	1.6	0
Chestnuts-shelled	2 Tbsp	53	0.8	7.3	0.5	1.6	124	0	0.06	0.06	0.16	0	0.09	0	0

Item	Amount	Calories	Protein grams	Cal-cium mg.	Iron mg.	Sod mg.	Potass mg.	A mcg.	Thia mg.	Ribo mg.	Nia mg.	C mg.	B₆ mg.	E mg.	Folic Acid mg.
English Walnuts shelled	2 Tbsp	172	4	27	0.9	T	123	8	0.09	0.04	0.25	0.5	0.2	6	2
Filberts-shelled	2 Tbsp	173	3.4	57	0.9	0.5	192	0	0.17	0	0.25	T	0.15	7.6	17
Peanuts															
shelled, whole	2 Tbsp	159	7.1	19.7	0.6	1.4	192	0	0.09	0.04	4.7	0	0	0	0
roasted, salted	2 Tbsp	159	7	20	0.6	114	183	0	0.09	0.04	4.7	0	0	0	0
Pecans-shelled	2 Tbsp	187	2.5	19.8	0.7	T	164	35	0.23	0.04	0.25	T	0.05	5.4	5
Pinenuts-shelled	2 Tbsp	173	3.5	2.8	1.4	0	0	10	0.35	0.07	1.26	T	0	0	0
Pistachio Nuts															
shelled	2 Tbsp	162	5.3	35.6	2	275	0	62	0.18	0	0.38	0	0	0	0
in the shell	2 Tbsp	81	2.6	17.8	1	132	0	31	0.09	0	0.19	0	0	1.4	0
Walnuts-shelled	2 Tbsp	171	5.6	T	1.6	T	125	82	0.06	0.03	0.19	0	0	0.7	0
Water Chesnuts	2 Tbsp	17	0.3	0.8	0.1	4	105	0	0.03	0.04	0.21	0.8	0	0	0
Peanut Butter	1 Tbsp	94	4	9	0.3	97	100	0	0	0	0.14	0	0	0	0
Pizza:															
Cheese	1 slice	153	7.8	144	0.7	456	85	410	0.4	0.13	0.7	5	0	0	0
Individual Frozen															
Cheese	1 slice	179	6.9	114	0.7	472	83	320	0.04	0.12	0.7	4	0	0	0
Sausage	1 slice	157	5.2	11	0.8	488	113	380	0.06	0.08	1	6	0	0	0
Popcorn:															
plain	1 cup	23	0.8	1	0.2	T	0	0	0	0.01	0.1	0	0.01	0	0
with oil and salt	1 cup	41	0.9	1	0.2	175	0	0	0	0.01	0.2	0	0.01	0	0
Potato Sticks	1 cup	190	2.2	15	0.6	46	0	T	0.07	0.02	1.7	14	0	0	0

Pretzels	4 oz	442	11	25	1.7	1905	148	0	0.09	0.14	3.2	0	0	0	0
Salad Dressings:															
Roquefort	1 Tbsp	76	0.7	12	T	164	6	30	T	0.02	T	T	0	0	0
Roquefort-Low Cal	1 Tbsp	3	0.2	5	T	170	4	10	T	0.01	T	T	0	0	0
French	1 Tbsp	66	0.1	2	0.1	219	13	0	0	0	0	T	0	0	0
French-Low Cal	1 Tbsp	15	0.1	2	0.1	126	13	0	0	0	0	0	0	0	0
Italian	1 Tbsp	83	T	2	T	314	2	T	T	T	T	T	0	0	0
Italian-Low Cal	1 Tbsp	8	T	T	T	118	2	T	T	T	T	T	0	0	0
Mayonnaise	1 Tbsp	101	0.2	3	0.1	84	5	T	0.01	0.01	0	T	0	0	0
Russian	1 Tbsp	74	0.2	3	0.1	130	24	100	0.01	0.01	0.1	1	0	0	0
Thousand Island	1 Tbsp	80	0.1	2	0.1	112	18	50	T	0.01	0.1	T	0	0	0
Thousand Island-Low Cal	1 Tbsp	27	0.1	2	0.1	105	17	50	T	T	T	T	0	0	0
Sesame Seeds	1 cup	873	27.3	165	3.6	0	0	0	0.27	0.2	8.1	0	0	0	0
Soups:															
Cream of Asparagus	1 cup	65	2.4	26	0.7	984	120	310	0.05	0.1	0.7	0	0	0	0
Beef Bouillon	1 cup	31	5	T	0.5	782	130	T	T	0.2	1.2	0	0	0	0
Beef Noodle	1 cup	67	3.8	7	1	917	77	50	0.05	0.07	1	T	0	0	0
Chicken Consomme	1 cup	22	3.4	12	1.2	0	0	0	0.02	0.05	0	0	0	0	0
Cream of Chicken	1 cup	94	2.9	24	0.5	970	79	410	0.02	0.12	0.5	T	0	0	0
Cream of Mushroom	1 cup	134	2.4	41	0.5	955	98	70	0.02	0.05	0.7	0	0.12	0	0
Chicken Gumbo	1 cup	55	3.1	19	0.5	950	108	220	0.02	0.02	1.2	T	0	0	0
Chicken Noodle	1 cup	62	3.4	10	0.5	979	55	50	T	0.02	0.7	5	0	0	0
Chicken with Rice	1 cup	48	3.1	7	0.2	917	98	140	0.02	0.02	0.7	T	0	0	0
Chicken Vegetable	1 cup	76	4.2	17	0.5	1034	98	2160	0.05	0.05	1	0	0	0	0
Clam Chowder (Manhattan)	1 cup	81	2.2	34	1	938	184	880	0.02	0.02	1	0	0	0	0
Minestrone	1 cup	105	4.9	37	1	995	314	2350	0.07	0.05	1	0	0	0	0
Onion	1 cup	65	5.3	29	0.5	1051	103	T	T	0.02	1	0	0	0	0
Pea, Split	1 cup	145	8.6	29	1.5	941	0	440	0.25	0.15	1.5	1	0	0	0

Item	Amount	Calories	Protein grams	Calcium mg.	Iron mg.	Sod mg.	Potass mg.	A mcg.	Thia mg.	Ribo mg.	Nia mg.	C mg.	B6 mg.	E mg.	Folic Acid mg.
Tomato	1 cup	88	2	15	0.7	970	230	1000	0.05	0.05	1.2	12	0.1	0	0
Turkey Noodle	1 cup	79	4.3	14	0.7	998	77	190	0.05	0.05	1.2	T	0	0	0
Vegetable Beef	1 cup	78	5.1	23	0.7	1046	162	2700	0.05	0.05	1	T	0	0	0
Vegetarian Vegetable	1 cup	78	2.2	20	1	838	172	2940	0.05	0.05	1	0	0	0	0
Dehydrated Soups:															
Beef Noodle	1 cup	67	2.4	10	0.5	420	41	20	0.1	0.05	0.7	T	0	0	0
Chicken Noodle	1 cup	53	1.9	7	0.2	578	19	50	0.07	0.05	0.05	T	0	0	0
Chicken Rice	1 cup	48	1.2	7	T	622	10	T	T	T	T	0.2	0	0	0
Onion	1 cup	36	1.4	10	0.2	689	58	T	T	T	T	2	0	0	0
Pea	1 cup	123	7.6	20	2	796	294	50	0.15	0.15	1.5	T	0	0	0
Tomato Vegetable with Noodles	1 cup	65	1.4	7	0.2	1025	29	480	0.05	0.02	0.5	5	0	0	0
Soy Sauce	1 cup	12	1	15	0.9	1319	66	0	T	0.05	0.1	0	0	0	0
Spaghetti in Tomato Sauce with Cheese:															
homemade	1 cup	260	8.8	80	2.3	955	408	1080	0.25	0.18	2.3	13	0	0	0
canned	1 cup	345	10	73	5	1733	549	1680	0.64	0.5	8.2	18	0	0	0
Spaghetti with Meatballs and Tomato Sauce:															
homemade	1 cup	332	18.6	124	3.7	1009	665	1590	0.25	0.3	4	22	0	0	0
canned	1 cup	258	12.3	53	3.3	1220	245	1000	0.15	0.18	2.3	5	0	0	0
Sunflower Seeds (hulled)	1 cup	812	34.8	174	44	1334	70	2.84	0.33	7.8	1.8	19	0

Item	Amount	Calories	Protein grams	Calcium mg.	Iron mg.	Sod mg.	Potass mg.	A mcg.	Thia mg.	Ribo mg.	Nia mg.	C mg.	B6 mg.	E mg.	Folic Acid mg.
Tartar Sauce	1 Tbsp.	74	0.2	3	0.1	99	11	30	T	T	T	T	0	0	0
Yeast, Bakers	1 ounce	24	3.4	4	1.4	5	173		0.2	0.47	3.2	T	0	0	0

SUGARS, SWEETS AND DESSERTS

Item	Amount	Calories	Protein grams	Calcium mg.	Iron mg.	Sod mg.	Potass mg.	A mcg.	Thia mg.	Ribo mg.	Nia mg.	C mg.	B6 mg.	E mg.	Folic Acid mg.
Homemade Cakes:															
Angelfood Cake	1 slice	241	6.3	8	0.2	253	79	0	T	0.13	0.18	0	—	—	—
Boston Cream Pie	1 slice	312	5.2	69	0.5	192	92	216	0.03	0.11	0.21	T	—	—	—
Caramel Cake	1 slice	597	5.8	132	2.4	397	101	315	0.03	0.11	0.16	T	—	—	—
Chocolate Cake (iced)	1 slice	550	6.7	104	1.5	351	230	239	0.03	0.15	0.3	T	—	—	—
Chocolate Cupcake	1	162	2	31	0.4	103	68	70	0.01	0.04	0.1	T	—	—	—
Fruitcake	1 slice	57	0.7	11	0.4	24	74	20	0.02	0.02	0.1	T	—	—	—
Gingerbread (iced)	1 piece	362	3.9	51	0.3	269	66	134	0.02	0.07	0.02	T	—	—	—
Gingerbread (plain)	1 piece	283	3.5	50	0.3	233	61	132	0.02	0.07	0.16	T	—	—	—
Pound Cake	1 slice	142	1.7	6	0.2	33	18	80	0.01	0.03	0.1	0	—	—	—
White Cake (iced)	1 slice	587	5.2	75	0.2	366	91	173	0.02	0.09	0.16	T	—	—	—
Yellow Cake (iced)	1 slice	549	6.3	102	0.9	313	162	240	0.03	0.12	0.3	T	—	—	—
Cakes made from mixes:															
Angelfood Cake	1 slice	206	4.5	75	0.2	116	48	0	0.04	0.09	0.08	0	—	—	—
Coffee Cake	1 piece	139	2.7	26	0.7	185	47	69	0.08	0.07	0.6	T	—	—	—
Cupcakes (iced)	1	172	2.2	62	0.4	161	56	80	0.02	0.05	0.1	T	—	—	—

Item	Amount	Calories	Protein grams	Calcium mg.	Iron mg.	Sod mg.	Potass mg.	A mcg.	Thia mg.	Ribo mg.	Nia mg.	C mg.	B$_6$ mg.	E mg.	Folic Acid mg.
Devil's Food Cake	1 slice	469	6.1	82	1.1	363	180	208	0.04	0.11	0.41	T	—	—	—
Honey Spice Cake	1 slice	543	6.3	110	1.2	378	127	248	0.03	0.14	0.31	T	—	—	—
Marble Cake	1 slice	432	5.7	102	1.1	338	159	118	0.02	0.11	0.26	T	—	—	—
White Cake	1 slice	513	5.6	141	0.7	234	162	85	0.03	0.11	0.28	T	—	—	—
Yellow Cake	1 slice	467	5.7	126	0.8	314	151	194	0.03	0.11	0.27	T	—	—	—
Candy:															
Butterscotch	1 ounce	113	T	5	0.4	19	1	40	0	T	T	0	—	—	—
Candy Corn	1 ounce	91	T	4	0.3	53	1	0	T	T	T	0	—	—	—
Caramels	1 ounce	113	1.1	42	0.4	64	54	T	0.01	0.05	0.1	T	—	—	—
Chocolate:															
Bittersweet	1 ounce	135	2.2	16	1.4	1	174	10	0.01	0.05	0.3	0	—	—	—
Milk	1 ounce	147	2.2	65	0.3	27	109	80	0.02	0.1	0.1	T	—	—	—
Semisweet	1 ounce	144	1.2	9	0.7	1	92	10	T	0.02	0.1	T	—	—	—
Chocolate Coated															
Almonds	1 ounce	161	3.5	58	0.8	17	155	T	0.03	0.15	0.5	T	—	—	—
Coconut	1 ounce	124	0.8	14	0.3	56	47	0	0.01	0.02	0.1	0	—	—	—
Fudge, Peanuts and Caramel	1 ounce	123	2.2	51	0.4	58	85	T	0.05	0.06	0.5	T	—	—	—
Peanuts	1 ounce	119	3.5	25	0.3	13	107	T	0.08	0.04	1.6	T	—	—	—
Raisins	1 ounce	101	1.3	36	0.6	15	143	36	0.02	0.05	0.1	T	—	—	—
Fudge (Chocolate)	1 ounce	122	1.1	29	0.4	65	55	T	0.01	0.04	0.1	0	—	—	—
Gumdrops	1 ounce	98	T	2	0.1	10	1	0	0	T	T	0	—	—	—
Jellybeans	1 ounce	101	T	3	0.3	3	T	0	0	T	T	0	—	—	—
Peanut Brittle	1 ounce	119	1.6	10	0.7	9	43	0	0.05	0.01	1	0	—	—	—

Food	Amount													
Cookies:														
Assorted Sandwich Type	1	55	0.57	4	0.08	41	8	9	T	T	T	1	—	—
Brownies with Nuts	1	97	1.3	8	0.4	50	38	40	0.04	0.02	0.1	T	—	—
Chocolate Chip (homemade)	1	52	0.5	5	0.2	35	12	10	0.01	0.01	0.1	T	—	—
Chocolate Chip (commercial)	1	50	0.57	4	0.2	42	14	13	T	0.01	0.04	T	—	—
Fig Bars	1	50	0.5	11	0.15	35	28	15	T	0.1	0.05	O	—	—
Macaroon	1	90	1	5	0.15	7	88	0	0.01	0.03	0.1	T	—	—
Oatmeal-Raisin	1	60	0.8	3	0.04	16	48	8	0.02	0.01	0.75	O	—	—
Peanut Sandwich	1	80	1.2	5	0.1	21	21	25	T	0.01	0.35	3	—	—
Sugar Wafer	1	17	0.17	1	0.01	7	2	5	T	T	0.02	T	—	—
Vanilla Wafer	1	14	0.16	1	0.01	8	2	4	T	T	0.01	O	—	—
Danish Pastry (Plain)	1	480	8.4	57	1	415	127	353	0.08	0.17	0.9	T	—	—
Pies:														
Apple	1 piece	302	2.6	9	0.4	355	94	40	0.02	0.02	0.5	1	—	—
Banana	1 piece	252	7.5	1	0.2	231	290	T	0.15	0.3	1	—	—	0.45
Blueberry	1 piece	286	2.8	13	0.7	316	77	40	0.02	0.02	0.4	4	—	—
Cherry	1 piece	308	3.1	17	0.4	359	124	520	0.07	0.02	0.6	T	—	—
Coconut Custard	1 piece	268	6.8	107	0.8	282	186	260	0.07	0.22	0.3	0	—	—
Lemon Meringue	1 piece	268	3.9	15	0.5	296	53	180	0.3	0.08	0.2	3	—	—
Mince	1 piece	320	3	33	1.2	529	210	T	0.08	0.05	0.5	1	—	—
Peach	1 piece	300	3	12	0.6	316	176	860	0.02	0.05	8	4	—	—
Pecan	1 piece	431	5.3	48	2.9	228	127	160	0.16	0.07	0.3	T	—	—
Pumpkin	1 piece	241	4.6	58	0.6	244	182	2810	0.03	0.11	0.6	T	—	—
Puddings (made from commercial mix with milk)	1 cup	322	8.8	265	0.8	335	354	340	0.05	0.39	0.3	2	—	—
Sherbert	1 cup	259	1.7	31	T	19	42	120	0.02	0.06	T	4	—	—

Item	Amount	Calories	Protein grams	Cal-cium mg.	Iron mg.	Sod mg.	Potass mg.	A mcg.	Thia mg.	Ribo mg.	Nia mg.	C mg.	B6 mg.	E mg.	Folic Acid mg.
Artichoke	1 heart	20	4.3	78	1.7	46	458	230	0.11	0.03	1.1	12	0	0	0
Asparagus spears:															
canned, green	1 cup	51	5.8	46	4.6	571	402	1940	0.15	0.24	0.2	36	0.13	0	23
canned, white	1 cup	53	5.1	39	2.4	571	339	190	0.12	0.15	1.7	36	0.08	0	0
cooked, boiled whole	1 cup	36	4	38	1.1	2	329	1620	0.29	0.32	2.5	47	0	0	0
frozen, cooked	1 cup	44	6.1	42	2.1	2	452	1480	0.3	0.27	2.1	49	0.39	0	0
Beans, boiled & cut french style	1 cup	31	2	62	0.8	5	189	675	0.09	0.11	0.6	14	0.11	0	0
Beans, canned without pork	1 cup	300	16	170	5	844	670	150	0.18	0.1	1.6	4	0	0	0
Beans, Kidney:															
canned	1 cup	225	14	73	4.5	8	660	T	0.13	0.10	1.5	0	0	0	0
cooked	1 cup	300	20	95	6	7.5	850	T	0.28	0.15	1.8	0	1.1	0	0
Beans, Lima															
canned, drained	1 cup	220	12	64	3.6	540	510	436	0.06	0.12	1.2	14	0	0	0
cooked	1 cup	178	12	75	4	1.6	675	448	0.29	0.16	2.0	29	0	0	0
frozen	1 cup	188	12	56	4.2	160	681	368	0.12	0.08	1.6	27	0.27	0	0
Beans, White:															
raw	1 cup	680	44	288	15.6	38	2392	0	1.3	0.44	4.8	0	0	0	0
cooked	1 cup	224	15	95	5.1	13	790	0	0.27	0.13	1.3	0	0	2	0

Beans, yellow or wax:															
canned	1 cup	48	2.8	90	3	472	190	200	0.06	0.1	0.6	10	0.08	0	5
cooked	1 cup	22	1.4	50	0.6	3	243	250	0.08	0.1	0.8	26	0.8	0	0
frozen, cooked	1 cup	54	2.4	70	1.4	2	320	200	0.14	0.16	0.8	12	0.15	0	0
Beansprouts, ming:															
cooked	1 cup	28	3.2	17	0.9	4	156	20	0.09	0.1	0.7	6	0	0	0
raw	1 cup	21	2.2	42	0.8	3	134	12	0.08	0.08	0.5	12	0	0	0
Beets:															
canned	1 cup	62	1.6	32	1.2	392	276	34	0.02	0.04	0.2	6	0	0	0
cooked	1 cup	54	1.8	24	0.8	72	244	34	0.06	0.06	0.6	10	0	0	0
Broccoli:															
cooked	1 cup	39	4.7	132	1.2	15	400	3900	0.09	0.18	0.8	135	0	0	0
raw	1-5½" stalk	32	3.6	103	1.1	15	328	2500	0.01	0.23	9	113	0.2	1.9	2
Brussels Sprouts															
cooked	1 cup	54	6.3	48	1.5	15	409	780	0.12	0.21	1.2	130	0	4.3	0
Cabbage:															
cooked	1 cup	33	1.8	22	0.5	23	272	216	0.07	0.07	0.5	70	0	0	0
red, raw	1 cup	31	2	42	0.8	26	268	40	0.09	0.06	0.4	61	0	0	0
Carrot:															
cooked	1 cup	47	1.4	50	0.9	50	333	15750	0.08	0.08	0.8	9	0	0	0
raw	1 large	42	1.1	37	0.7	47	341	11000	0.06	0.05	0.6	8	0.15	0.5	8
Cauliflower:															
cooked	1 cup	28	2.9	26	0.9	11	258	80	0.11	0.1	0.8	69	0	0	0
raw	1 cup	27	2.7	25	1.1	13	295	60	0.11	0.1	0.7	78	0.32	0.15	31

Item	Amount	Calories	Protein grams	Calcium mg.	Iron mg.	Sod mg.	Potass mg.	A mcg.	Thia mg.	Ribo mg.	Nia mg.	C mg.	B₆ mg.	E mg.	Folic Acid mg.
Celery:															
cooked	1 cup	18	1	39	0.3	110	200	388	0.03	0.4	0.4	8	0	0	0
raw	1 stalk	7	0.4	16	0.1	50	136	110	0.01	0.01	0.1	4	0.03	0.25	4
Chickpeas	1 cup	720	41	300	14	62	1600	100	0.62	0.3	4	0	1.1	5.1	2
Coleslaw (with mayonnaise)	1 cup	173	1.6	53	0.5	144	239	190	0.06	0.06	0.4	T	0	0	0
Collard Greens (cooked)	1 cup	150	3.2	853	3.6	0	1188	35380	0.5	0.9	5.4	345	0	0	0
Cucumber	½ medium size	8	0.5	13	0.6	3	80	125	0.15	0.2	0.1	6	0.02	0	0
Eggplant (cooked)	½ cup	19	1	11	0.6	1	150	10	0.5	0.4	0.5	3	0	0	0
Kale (cooked)	½ cup	19	2.1	90	0.8	29	148	4956	T	T	0.7	62	0	0	0
Lentils	1 cup	212	15.6	50	4.2	0	498	40	0.14	0.12	1.2	0	1.2	5	0
Lettuce (Iceberg, NY and Great Lakes)	1 cup	28	2.4	70	4	18	528	1980	0.12	0.12	0.6	16	0.01	1	23
Mushrooms	4 large/10 small	28	2.7	6	0.8	15	414	T	0.01	0.46	4.2	3	0.14	0.1	3
Okra (cooked)	8-9 pods	29	2	92	0.5	2	174	490	0.13	0.18	0.9	20	0	0	0
Olives	10	45	0.5	24	0.6	926	21	120	0	0	0	0	0.006	0	0

Food	Measure														
Onion:															
cooked	1 cup	61	2.5	50	0.8	15	231	80	0.06	0.06	0.04	15	0	0	0
raw	1 cup	65	26	46	0.9	17	267	70	0.05	0.07	0.3	17	0.22	0.4	20
Parsley	1 cup	26	2.2	122	3.7	27	436	5100	0.07	0.16	0.7	103	0.09	1.8	30
Peas:															
canned	1 cup	99	5	30	2.5	353	144	675	135	74	1.4	13	0	0	0
cooked	1 cup	107	8.1	35	2.7	2	294	210	420	165	3.5	30	0	0	0
frozen	1 cup	102	7.7	28	2.8	172	202	900	405	135	2.6	20	0	0	0
raw	1 cup	105	7.9	33	2.4	2	395	800	438	172	3.6	34	0	0	0
Peas & Carrots (frozen)	4 ounces	60	3.6	28	1.3	95	178	10545	0.22	0.08	1.5	9	0	0	0
Peppers:															
Green, raw	1 pepper	36	2	15	1.1	21	349	690	0.13	0.13	0.8	210	0.52	1.4	20
Hot Chili	1 cup	51	2.2	22	1.2	0	0	23500	0.02	0.22	1.5	71	0	0	0
Sweet Green (cooked)	1 pepper	29	1.6	15	0.8	14	238	690	0.1	0.11	0.7	T	0.41	0	0
Pickles:															
Dill	1 pickle	7	0.5	17	0.7	928	130	70	T	0.01	T	4	0.04	0	0
Sour	1 pickle	7	0.3	11	2.1	879	0	70	T	0.01	T	5	0.04	0	0
Sweet	1 pickle	22	0.1	2	0.2	0	0	10	T	T	T	1	0.02	0	0
Pickle Relish	1 cup	338	1.2	49	2	1744	0	0	0	0	0	0	0	0	0
Potatoes:															
baked	1	145	4	14	1.1	6	782	T	0.15	0.07	2.7	31	0	0	0
boiled	1	173	4.8	16	1.4	7	926	T	0.2	0.09	3.4	36	0	0.5	0
french fried	¼ pound	311	5	17	1.5	7	967	T	0.15	0.09	3.5	24	0	0	0
frozen, french fried	10	110	1.8	5	0.9	2	326	T	0.07	0.01	1.3	11	0	0	0

Item	Amount	Calories	Protein grams	Cal-cium mg.	Iron mg.	Sod mg.	Potass mg.	A mcg.	Thia mg.	Ribo mg.	Nia mg.	C mg.	B6 mg.	E mg.	Folic Acid mg.
mashed in milk scalloped au gratin with cheese	1 cup	137	4.4	50	0.8	632	548	40	0.17	0.11	2.1	21	0	0	0
	1 cup	355	13	311	1.2	1095	750	780	0.15	0.29	2.2	25	0	0	0
Potato Chips	10 chips	113	1.1	8	0.4	226	0	T	0.04	0.01	1	3	T	0	1
Potato Salad (homemade without eggs)	¼ pound	112	3	36	0.7	599	362	160	0.09	0.08	1.3	13	0	0	0
Radishes	1 small	2	0.1	3	0.1	2	32	1	0.003	0.003	0.03	3	T	0	T
Rutabaga (cooked)	1 cup	60	1.5	100	0.5	7	284	940	0.1	0.1	1.4	44	0	0	0
Sauerkraut	1 cup	42	2.4	85	1.2	1755	329	120	0.07	0.09	0.5	33	0.29	0	0
Soybeans (cooked)	1 cup	177	15	90	4	0	0	990	0.47	0.2	1.8	26	0.3	0	892
Soybean curd (Tofu)	3½ ounces	72	7.8	128	1.9	7	42	0	0.06	0.03	0.1	0	0.3	0	363
Spinach: boiled canned frozen, cooked	1 cup 1 cup 1 cup	42 44 48	5.4 4.8 5.8	166 212 210	4 4.6 5	90 424 98	582 454 724	14300 14400 16200	0.12 0.04 0.16	0.26 0.22 0.28	1 0.6 0.5	50 26 56	0.34 0.15 0.4	0 0 0	3 42 0
Squash: acorn, baked	1 cup	126	3.6	56	1.6	2		8400	0.1	0.26	1.4	26	0	0	0

Food	Measure													
acorn, boiled	1 cup	83	2.9	45	1.7	2	750	2700	0.1	0.25	0.16	20	0	0	0
summer, cooked	1 cup	28	1.8	50	0.8	2	282	780	0.1	0.16		20	0	0	0
winter, cooked	1 cup	95	3	50	1.2	25	645	8750	0.1	0.25		20	0	0	0
winter, frozen and cooked	1 cup	72	2.4	50	52	2	414	7800	0.06	1.42	1	16	0.4	0	0
Succotash, frozen and cooked	½ pound	211	9.6	30	2.3	86	558	680	0.2	0.12	3	14	0.4	0	0
Sweet Potatoes:															
baked	1	161	2.4	46	1	14	342	9230	0.1	0.08	0.8	26	0	0	0
boiled	1	172	2.6	48	1.1	15	367	11940	0.14	0.09	0.9	26	0	0	0
candied	2 halves	168	1.3	37	0.9	42	190	6300	0.06	0.04	0.4	10	0	0	0
canned	1 small	108	2	25	0.8	48	200	7800	0.05	0.04	0.6	14	0	0	14
Tomatoes:															
canned	1 cup	42	2	12	1	260	424	1800	0.1	0.06	1.4	34	0	0	0
paste	1 cup	215	8.9	71	9.2	100	2237	8650	0.52	0.31	8.1	128	0	0	0
puree	1 cup	97	4.2	32	4.2	1000	1060	4000	0.22	0.12	3.5	82	0	0	14
ripe	1 medium	33	1.6	20	0.8	4	366	1350	0.09	0.06	1	34	0.22	0.8	
Tomato Catsup	1 Tbsp.	16	0.3	3	0.1	156	54	210	0.01	0.01	0.2	2	0	0	0
Tomato Chili Sauce	1 Tbsp.	16	0.4	3	0.1	201	56	210	0.01	0.01	0.2	2	0	0	0
Tomato Juice:															
can or bottle	1 cup	46	2.2	17	2.2	486	552	1940	0.12	0.07	1.9	39	0.5	0	0
cocktail	1 cup	51	1.7	24	2.2	486	537	1940	0.12	0.05	1.5	36	0.4	0	0
low sodium	1 cup	46	1.9	17	2.2	7	549	1940	0.12	0.07	1.7	39	0.4	0	0
Turnips (cooked)	1 cup	34	1.2	53	0.6	51	282	T	0.06	0.08	0.5	33	0	0	0
Turnip Greens (cooked)	1 cup	30	3.3	276	1.7	0	0	9450	0.23	0.36	0.9	103	0	0	0

Item	Amount	Calories	Protein grams	Cal-cium mg.	Iron mg.	Sod mg.	Potass mg.	A mcg.	Thia mg.	Ribo mg.	Nia mg.	C mg.	B$_6$ mg.	E mg.	Folic Acid mg.
Vegetable Juice Cocktail	1 cup	41	2.2	29	1.2	484	535	1690	0.12	0.07	1.9	22	0	0	0
Vegetables, mixed	1 cup	116	5.8	46	2.4	96	348	9010	0.22	0.13	2	15	0	0	0
Yams (cooked)	1 cup	210	4.8	8	1.2	0	0	T	0.18	0.08	1.2	18	0	0	0

Index

Accutane, 164
Acetylcholine, 185–87
Acne, Vitamin A and, 164
Acrodermatitis enteropathica, 238
Addison's disease (pernicious anemia), 126, 129, 141
Adolescents, *see* Teenagers
Adriamycin, 175
Aging
  chromium and, 61
  manganese and, 65, 253
  and nutrient absorption, 51
  selenium and, 65, 259
  vitamin E and, 171
Agricultural methods, 30–31
Albee with C, 76, 84
Albee C-800, 76, 84
Albee C-800 plus Iron, 86
Albinism, 246
Alcohol, 36
  vitamin C and, 148, 152, 276
  and zinc, 238–39
Alcoholism
  choline and liver damage from, 187–88
  folic acid and, 138
  supplements and, 50–51, 109
  vitamin B_1 and, 95–96
Alkaline phosphatase, 239
Allopurinol, 255, 281
Alpha tocopherol, 171–72
Aluminum hydroxide antacids, 220
Alzheimer's disease, 187
American Psychiatric Association, 58
Amine structure, 7

Aminosalicylic acid (PAS), 130, 148, 275, 276
Amitryptilline, 103
Amygdalin, 195
Anemia
  copper deficiency and, 247
  differentiation of, 138, 233
  folic acid and, 130, 138, 139
  hemolytic, 175
  iron-deficiency (hypochromic micro-cytic), 232–33, 269
  megaloblastic, 46, 130, 138
  pernicious (Addison's disease), 126, 129, 141
  from pyridoxine deficiency, 120
  in vitamin C deficiency, 143, 146
Antacids, 220, 281
Aquasol A, 11
Aquasol E, 11
Anticoagulants, *see* Oral anticoagulant drugs
Antidepressant drugs, 276
Apresoline, *see* Hydralazine
Arachadonic acid, 198
Arsenic, 12, 261
Arthritis, copper and, 248
Ascorbic acid, *see* vitamin C
Athletes, 48–49, 68, 178
Avidin, 132

Baldness, 79–80
Barbiturates, 169, 274, 279
"Basic Four" food groups, 34–36
Bedsores, 152
Beminal 500, 76, 84

347

351

357